VEGAN FREAK
BEING VEGAN IN A NON-VEGAN WORLD

VERSION 2.0: REVISED, EXPANDED, AND UPDATED

VEGAN FREAK
BEING VEGAN IN A NON-VEGAN WORLD

VERSION 2.0: REVISED, EXPANDED, AND UPDATED

Bob Torres, PhD

Jenna Torres, PhD

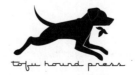

tofu hound press

DISCLAIMER: Though this book has been thoroughly researched, the opinions herein are offered for educational and entertainment purposes only. Before any change in diet, readers should consult a physician or nutritionist. Although the authors and publisher have made every effort to ensure the accuracy and completeness of information contained in this book, we assume no responsibility for errors, inaccuracies, omissions, or any inconsistency herein.

Vegan Freak: Being Vegan in a Non-Vegan World, 2nd Edition
© Bob Torres and Jenna Torres 2010
This edition © PM Press 2010

ISBN: 978-1-60486-015-3

Library of Congress Control Number: 2008934203

Cover design by John Yates
Interior design by Ida Fong

10 9 8 7 6 5 4 3 2 1

PM Press
PO Box 23912
Oakland, CA 94623
www.pmpress.org

Printed in the USA on recycled paper.

To Mole, Emmy, Michi, Taco, and Spike,
who remind us every day why we're vegan.

To our parents, who have always been there for us.

ACKNOWLEDGEMENTS

THE SUPPORT OF MANY PEOPLE HAVE HELPED US TO MAKE THIS BOOK WHAT IT IS:

Thanks to Ramsey and everyone else at PM Press for being incredibly patient with us and our delays, and for helping us to get this book to print. Thanks to Romy Ruukel for her deft copy editing, and to John Yates for the brilliant new cover. Thanks also go to Alli Dunlap for all her help with the manuscript and with Tofu Hound Press, and to Ida Fong for her wonderful design work and for putting up with our forever changing production schedule. (Don't worry: we love you too, Mr. Fong.)

We owe abundant thanks to the many of you who sent us feedback on the first edition of *Vegan Freak*, all our freakies on the forums, and all our devoted podcast listeners. Thanks for all the words of encouragement, the great voicemails and emails (both hilarious and thought-provoking), and for helping us to create a community of vegans where people don't feel so alone.

Gary Francione and Anna Charlton have been working tirelessly for years to promote nonviolent vegan education while simultaneously developing what we believe to be the only sensible articulation of the moral and ethical necessity of granting animals personhood. Their years of writing, teaching, and speaking on these issues have created a sensible, non-violent movement for the abolition of animal exploitation where none previously existed, and their ideas have utterly transformed the ways that we approach our own work. As if redefining an entire field of study weren't enough, Gary and Anna are also extraordinarily generous with their time, energy, and advice, and we count them among our very best friends.

As in the first edition of the book, our cat Michi once again helped during production by sitting on Jenna's keyboard and blocking her monitor, while the new kittens Taco and Spike also got into the game by typing, trying to chew on our copies of the first edition of *Vegan Freak*, running off with all of our pens and pencils, darting around the house like crazy, and being distractingly cute. Our dogs Mole and Emmy watched over our offices and kept us company as we wrote, barked like crazy at anyone who dared come close to the elite fortress, and made sure we got out for a walk every day.

We also can't forget Ida and Richard and Hy and Ceile for being great people and awesome friends. Hy and Ceile, we miss you and thank you for being there for us through thick and thin. Ida and Richard, we always know we can count on you to go out for awesome vegan food, talk about crazy shit and to commiserate about all manner of things. You all have always been kind, supportive, and understanding, and we thank you profusely. Bob also wishes to thank Dr. Don Haupt for his support. Don: I know you think this veganism stuff is insane, but at least we agree on stand-up comedians, so all is not lost. Jenna wants to thank Doug Nelson and Scott Meadows for being incredibly accommodating about her veganism and for even offering to go to a vegan restaurant for dinner!

And finally, thanks to our parents — Bob, Debbie, Keith, and Sandy — and to Zach and Carly for always being so enthusiastic about our book, for being supportive and putting up with all our weirdness, and for always making us awesome vegan food.

TABLE OF CONTENTS

PREFACE TO VERSION 2.0

BACK IN THE EARLY SPRING OF 2005 when we began floating the idea of writing the first edition of *Vegan Freak*, some prominent folks in the animal rights movement did their best to dissuade us. "Other books already do this," they said, or, "The movement doesn't need a book like this right now," or, "Why not devote your energy to something else?" Being the ever-stubborn anti-authoritarians that we are, we ignored the doomsayers and forged ahead anyway. We figured that if we felt like there was a hole in the existing offerings, other people must feel as we did, and so, with little fanfare, the first version of *Vegan Freak* was published in 2005. At the time, we figured we'd meet real success if we could find a thousand like-minded souls to buy a copy.

We've long since surpassed our initial expectations — and, as it turns out, the naysayers were wrong, too. *Vegan Freak* did strike a chord with many of you, and slowly, we've grown the idea from the book into a community of people from around the world who embrace veganism in their everyday lives. Linked together through forums and an online radio show at veganfreakradio.com, the community that grew out of the humble set of ideas from the first edition of this book has organized meet-ups all throughout the world, joined together for activism, and generally worked to support what is the first and most essential aspect of animal rights activism: going vegan. The community, the show, and the book have collectively helped thousands of people to go vegan and stay vegan, and, by any measure, that is the most important thing to have grown out of this effort. We hope to keep that momentum going through the second edition, too, and to help to build something even larger and more powerful: a vegan social movement that seeks to abolish the exploitation and commodification of animals.

Since writing the first edition of this book, our ideas and perspectives have matured a bit. Looking back, there's a lot that we're proud of, but there's also a great deal more that we think we could do more effectively, not only to produce a better book, but to get more people to go vegan and stay vegan. This fully revised (and mostly rewritten book) sets out to rectify some of those original holes in our approach, while retaining at least some of the generally irreverent and personal character of the first version of *Vegan Freak*.

Normally, in the publishing industry, doing a second edition requires about 20 percent of the book to be rewritten. When we were approached by the fine folks at PM Press to do our second edition, we told them 20 percent wouldn't be enough for us to feel like we'd done work we could stand behind. To make the book feel fresh, to adjust it to our current thinking, and to give you the best possible bang for your buck (or pound, or yen, or whatever) we decided that we'd do an almost complete rewrite. What you're holding in your hands presently is the result of that rewrite. We hope you will enjoy the book, read it with an open mind, and think carefully about the ideas that we put forth. They stem from our years of writing, speaking, and teaching about these ideas at the university level. This book is, in many more ways, a more mature book, both in tone and in outlook. Our theoretical and practical perspectives have come a long way, and we try to impart some of that to you in this new edition.

That said, there will always be critics — as there should be. No book is perfect, and every book is, by its nature, partial and limited by the experience and knowledge of its authors. Nevertheless, as the cliché goes, everyone's a critic — mostly because it is easier to be one than to actually go to the trouble of writing something yourself. Still, the critiques did not go unnoticed, and we've tried to address some of them in this new edition. Some people said our book was "smug" and "not funny." Well, this version is even more smug and probably even less funny. One particularly trenchant and perspicacious critic on Amazon.com whose words can still bring a tear to the eyes of these hardened, cynical authors wrote that the first edition of this book "like, used too many other books," because we, like, cited our sources, and gave credit to people whose ideas we used. In this book, we continue in that sad and, like, totally unnecessary tradition of crediting our intellectual forbearers. Sorry, high-school and college-aged plagiarizers everywhere: you may not count us among your ranks, mostly because we're much older than all of you. Oh, and because we cite our sources.

Our first book also included several small digs at crusty, Volvo-driving, middle-aged leftover hippie-types, many of whom, we suggested, took themselves far too seriously and had a poor sense of humor. Indeed, we were proven right on both counts when many of these said middle-aged granola-types wrote grumpy letters to us about how they did have a sense of humor — damnit! — but that we just needed to respect our elders. In this edition, we direct most of our mocking scorn towards the hipster scourge that has subsumed the identity and originality of untold millions under cans of Pabst Blue Ribbon, fixed-gear bikes, and DIY-knit iPod cozies.

We also have a thing or two to say about certain celebrities, though we do take a dig here and there at the self-absorbed gray-hairs who still remember Woodstock with fondness. We figure that you all have found yourselves and aligned your chakras by now, so a little good-natured ribbing from two opinionated fools in their mid-30s should probably not harsh your mellow too much. Put on some Enya or Joni Mitchell, do some "aromatherapy," and relax. After all, we're sure your guru in India would tell you that light-heartedness is good for the soul. (Actually, we're pretty sure your guru in India would tell you whatever you wanted to hear if you paid him enough.)

Finally, some people suggested that the first edition was too mean. Yet others said it was too nice. It comes down to this: no book can be everything to everyone, and any book that tries to be is usually unmitigated crap. For those of you who said we were too mean: in this edition, we could have served up cloying, warmed-over spoonfuls of feel-good, ethically-ambiguous pap about the wonders of cage-free eggs or about how you are a delicate and fragile being who has to have compassion first and foremost for yourself. On the other end of the spectrum, for those who said we were too nice: we could also easily have written a book about how you should channel your inner punk, tell people to fuck themselves and flip over the table anytime anyone — including your dear, old 85-year-old grandmother — offers you a non-vegan food item. But we end up at neither end of this particular spectrum, and instead chart what we see as an honest and ethically rigorous course throughout the book. Our ultimate goal is to put together the ethical and moral theory of the abolitionist vegan movement with everyday practice, and to do so with a sense of humor. We never apologize for our ethics, and a big part of our book is getting you, as a vegan or potential vegan, not to apologize for yours, either.

When it comes down to it, if we spend too much time listening to the critics, we never listen to ourselves, and we probably never would have written this book. As Virgil said, "Fortune favors the bold." We agree, and we hope you can convince you to take bold steps towards living as a proud vegan as you work through this book.

— Bob Torres & Jenna Torres
August 2009

"The world only goes forward because of those who oppose it"

— Goethe —

CHAPTER 1

VEGAN AND FREAKY

"IF YOU'RE GOING TO LEAVE WITH ANYONE TODAY, I'D LIKE TO SEE YOU LEAVE WITH HER."

The "her" in this case was Emmy, a then-eighteen-month-old medium-sized black shepherd mix, with a puffy, wild tail, and a calm but confident demeanor. She was, in every way that we could tell, a sweet and gentle dog, which is why what the director of the animal shelter told us came as a huge shock.

"She's been here a year, and she really just needs to be in a loving home. Don't get the wrong idea: she's a wonderful dog — we love her! She's friendly and house-trained, and great around cats. We just can't seem to adopt her out because she is black."

Naive as we were at the time, we'd not known about what's called "Black Dog Syndrome," the problem where black dogs are adopted at much lower rates because people have some kind of baseless fear about black dogs being more aggressive, or simply because black dogs don't match their furnishings or something. Whatever the ridiculous reason, it was apparently why a dog as sweet as Emmy had been living in a shelter for a year. At any other shelter that euthanized animals, Emmy would have been killed within weeks; yet, when we arrived at the local no-kill shelter that day, she was every bit the confident, scrappy, and happy little mutt that we've come to know her as in the years we lived with her. Full of vigor, and really just ready to get out of her kennel at the pound, Emmy came home with us. We had the room and the resources, and we were only too happy to take in another dog. Emmy was going to be part of our family.

On the way home in the car, it didn't take Emmy long to warm up to us. Almost immediately, she curled up on Jenna's lap — quite a feat for a dog who weighs sixty pounds, but it can be done — and from that moment onward, it was as though Emmy had nominated us as her people. Our common bond with her has grown stronger and stronger everyday since, and like all of the other animals with whom we live, Emmy is part of our family. At breakfast every morning, Emmy curls up at our feet under the table, and we'll occasionally slip her crust from our toast, or maybe a little chunk of banana, food that she always takes carefully and oh-so-gently, as if she might crush it if she weren't careful. Every night, Emmy stretches out at the foot of our bed (probably because one of our cats often sleeps in her bed, but that's another story). And every day when we write, Emmy is there to keep us company, with the nudge of a cold nose on the arm when our normal walk time rolls around.

It is probably clear by now, but we love Emmy dearly, just as we love our goofy, excitable, and playful lab Mole, our grass-munching, oversized eighteen-pound kitty Michi, and our two newest additions to the family, Spike and Taco, little kitten-brothers who came to us through a foster family. The little family of non-humans with whom we spend so much of our time has taught us a lot about what it means to be human, and what it means to love and be loved unconditionally. They've also taught us a lot about what it means to be non-human, and in doing so, they've helped us to overcome a lot of the hubris and pride that have colored our relations with animals in the past. In the years that we've been fortunate enough to share our lives with these non-human family members, we've come to know them to be as individual as any of us humans, if not more so. Long ago, we stopped thinking of them as "only animals" and have instead recognized how they simply possess a different set of skills and attributes than we humans do. Appreciating our animal family meant fully appreciating these differences.

As we began to evolve into this consciousness about the animals with whom we lived, we began to think critically and carefully about other animals, particularly the ones who died unnecessarily on a daily basis, only to end up on our plates as food. It doesn't take a great logical or emotional leap to wonder if these billions upon billions of animals were every bit as desirous for companionship and freedom as the dogs and cats with whom we shared our lives. Having taken one of his bachelor's degrees in agricultural science, Bob knew cows and pigs and chickens who responded by name, who recognized their "keepers," and reacted excitedly when they came to visit. These same animals were obviously happy when they were with their families and saddened when separated from those they felt companionship with. If pigs, cattle, chickens, sheep, and other animals were so much like the animals so many of us live with, the question for us was a simple one: what made pigs, cattle, chickens, and sheep so different from dogs and cats such that we killed one for food and cuddled with another on the couch?

Once we were honest with ourselves, the answer was surprisingly simple: there really isn't any difference that matters when it comes to the essential aspects of how we'd all like to be treated. In so far as all of those animals are sentient and have clear psychological, lasting, and subjective experiences of reality, their imprisonment, slaughter, and outright exploitation are no more just than the imprisonment, slaughter, or outright exploitation of our dogs, our cats, or even of any of us members of the human community. Being the well-socialized beings that we are, we all have little internal voices with answers at the ready for times like this. Like a good little cop for the existing order of things, the brain sounds the klaxons, puts up "DO NOT ENTER" signs, and spits back familiar yet comfortable responses. "Animals are ours to use." "They were brought into existence to serve us." "They're not as smart as we are." "They're tasty." "What would we eat if we didn't eat animals?" "If I didn't eat animal protein, I might die, or at least I'd look like some skinny-ass, pale vegan." Unfortunately for the billions of animals a year that die for no other good reason than the fact that we humans like to eat them, these are the scripts that we all have in our heads about the way the world operates; these ideas not only reflect the current order of things, they also espouse a sense of how many of us believe things should be.

Veganism as a process and as a way of life is all about asking you to rewrite those internal scripts to recognize the inherent worth of animals. Coming to this awareness is complex and at times frustrating, making ethical veganism a complex gift. We'd be lying to you if we said it was easy to buck thousands of years of tradition and to deny the received social and cultural wisdom that says that doing things the same old way is just fine. Running against history is never easy, and there are times when it sucks. Yet, if we're serious about justice and compassion, we must be serious about it for even what many would consider the least of us. In order to be consistent in our ideas of what constitutes equity, our notions of justice and compassion must expand outward to include non-human animals. As a vegan, or a soon-to-be-vegan, you will be at the forefront of this new and evolving cultural and social understanding. You will be the one who helps to right the thousands of years of wrongs. You will be the one who recognizes that the old way of doing things can't be the way we continue to do things. You will be one of the many to stand up and say enough.

Our goal is to help you along on this journey. When we first heard about veganism, we thought it was a bit nuts, too. We weren't sure that it was necessary, desirable, or even achievable, and we certainly weren't sure that we wanted to bother with going much beyond regular old vegetarianism. We weren't born into vegan families, and so we've come to this on our own terms. Though we have built up years of experience on the topic by teaching, writing, and speaking about it, we still clearly remember those first few fledgling weeks as proto-vegans, and we bring that awareness to what we're doing here. With measured doses of humor, logic, advice, and tough love, we'll help you to go vegan, or, if you're already vegan, we are going to encourage you to think about veganism in new ways that will reinvigorate the passion that got you to go vegan in the first place.

Vej-uns, VAYguns, and Vegans Oh My

"But you don't looooook like a VAY-gun."

Oh? And what does a VAY-gun look like? And what the hell is a VAY-gun anyway?

We've both heard this particular refrain — we never can decide if it is a compliment or an insult — on more occasions than we care to count. Why can't people just get the pronunciation right? We aren't VAY-guns or VEEJ-uns, we're vegans, you know, with a long "e," like if you say the letter "v" and

5

then add the word "gun" to it. Said correctly, the term "vegan" rhymes with the way a Canadian or American would say the name Tegan, as in half of the group Tegan and Sara. Vegan does not rhyme with "ray gun," though "ray gun" is a fabulous way to say the last name of the 40th president of the United States, given his penchant for space weaponry and lasers and shit like that.

To get back to the idea of neither of us looking like vegans, we begin to honestly wonder: just what kinds of absurd stereotypes are people walking around with in their heads to get them to say such a ridiculous thing out loud? On the few occasions when either of us have asked people what they meant and people are honest enough to answer us, we usually we get some kind of combination of answers that draw almost fully on misconceptions about vegans. To most people who even know what a vegan is — admittedly, less of a problem now than when we did the first edition of this book — one of a few different stereotypes springs to mind. The most predominant misconception that we hear is that vegans are dreadlocked, stinky hippies, endlessly fascinated with hemp, hemp seeds, hemp milk, and/or marijuana. To most people who think of vegans as hippies, we're clearly too busy chewing on granola and hanging out with the Rainbow Family in some national forest to really wrap our heads around how the world works. Some people think of vegans as impossibly skinny and malnourished, with yellow skin, thinning hair, and brittle nails because all we eat is tofu and apple juice. Yet others see vegans as judgmental, moralizing nut jobs who drive hybrid cars, endlessly lecture people on sustainability and "carbon footprints," buy shoes made out of recycled tires, and refuse to eat anything that casts a shadow (Admittedly, this stereotype may actually have some truth to it). Neither of us really fit any of the above stereotypes, so people probably get confused, and end up telling us that we don't look like VAY-guns.

The thing is, there are actually vegan hippies (shocker, right?). There are also vegans who are malnourished because they subsist only on hummus, cupcakes, potato chips, and Coke. And there are obviously vegans who are judgmental assholes — actually there are plenty of them in our experience. But there are also vegan writers (including at least one Nobel Prize winner), vegan chefs, vegan firefighters, vegan people in the military, vegan moms and dads, vegan teachers, vegan congressmen, and probably even vegan ninjas and pirates (for the record: we think ninjas are cooler than pirates). There are vegans who are, without a doubt, insane, and vegans who are the very definition of sanity and composure. There are punk vegans and skinny PBR-drinking hipster vegans with fixed-gear bikes who wear chunky black glasses and Goth vegan vampires. There are vegans in Vienna and Venezuela. There are vegans who look like your mom and dad and your sister and brother. The point is that vegans come from all walks of life, from all ages, all genders (female, male, transgender, and otherwise), all sexual orientations, all body sizes, all races, all income levels, all political orientations (though really, we wonder about conservative vegans), and many nationalities. Of course, if you don't actually know a vegan in real life, it is easy to let a stereotype constructed by the media give you all the details about how vegans look and act. Take it from the half of this dynamic writing duo with the Ph.D. in sociology: if nothing else, we humans are social creatures who value predictability, and that translates into us working most easily in generalities and their closely related cousin, the ever-dreaded stereotype. But as with all stereotypes, casting a single group under such a broad umbrella and making assumptions about people in that group is a troubling business, a business that is fraught with traps for the uninitiated and unfamiliar.

In this book, we need you to understand these stereotypes, because as you move more into veganism, you're going to have to confront them head-on, whether you like it or not. Ideally, we'll build a movement of people that is big enough, diverse enough, and vibrant enough so that we can begin to dismantle a bit of the wayward thinking about vegans, but in the meantime, you need to recognize that the stereotypes are out there. One of our primary goals is to give you some tools to deal with living with the ridiculous, unreal, and often bafflingly stupid expectations foisted upon you by unknowing friends, family, and others. It is like we vegans are some kind of exotic tribe that was recently discovered deep in the Amazonian jungle: people are unsure of what we eat, how we act, what we believe, and what we're all about. We wish people would just chill out already; we're not that foreign. We have the number zero; we understand how fire works; and we even have rudimentary technology. Granted, we are an odd and ragtag tribe that sometimes gets along and sometimes doesn't, but what unites us as a tribe of ethical vegans is our shared belief that eating and using animal products is wrong — otherwise, we just wouldn't be vegans. Just as people would probably misunderstand the habits and customs of the indigenous person from Amazonia regaled in feathers and face paint, they misunderstand our habits and customs and beliefs, too. So, regardless of how "normal" you are, in a world where consuming animal products is the norm, you're always going to be seen as the freak if you obviously and clearly refuse to take part in an act of consumption that is central to our everyday lives, our cultures, and even our very own personal identities.

To correct a misunderstanding that many people had about the first edition of this book before having even bothered to read it, we don't think that all vegans are freaks, and we don't think you have to be a freak to be a vegan. However, it is patently clear that if you consciously separate yourself from others through everyday choices about food and other aspects of your life, you're going to be viewed differently by those around you. This difference isn't something you should run from. On the contrary, you should embrace this freakdom, be at home with it, and fully own it, not only for your own sanity, but also for the efficacy of building a vegan social movement as a whole. This ownership of your vegan freakdom is also the first and most critical step towards keeping you a happy vegan and building genuine vegan community. Whether you're a new vegan or whether you've been a vegan for the last decade or more, recognizing this vital aspect of veganism is essential not only to your own long-term mental health but also to the long-term success of veganism as a community and movement of people who collectively decide say "enough already!" when it comes to the use and abuse of animals for human ends. It should go without saying that we wish being vegan were the most normal thing in the world, but at this point, we all should be honest with ourselves about the need to get more people to go vegan. As of this writing, there are more people in the United States who believe that they've had contact with extraterrestrials than there are people who are vegan.[1] This means that our approaches are only middling in their success, or the extraterrestrial biological entities are stepping things up in their plans for intergalactic domination, or, perhaps, both.

What Veganism Is

People are not only confused about what vegans look like — they're confused about what veganism really is. A great deal of the blame for this can be laid at the feet of wishy-washy, non-committal people who like the label "vegan" for whatever reason but who nevertheless do obviously non-vegan things like eat cheese "on occasion," or have meat "every once in a while." Many of these same so-called "vegans" also eat cage-free eggs, or organic meats on occasion because they absurd-ly believe these products to be somehow "less cruel," and somehow more acceptable. Let's just get this out there now, right at the start of the book, Michael Pollan and his localvore meat-eating sycophants be damned: being vegan means avoiding animal products to the greatest extent possible, not because of some conception of personal purity, but because ethical vegans live their politics every single day as a form of protest against the use and abuse of animals for human ends. Veganism is our way of expressing our anger — yes, our anger! — with the injustice perpetuated through industries and practices that exploit animals. As vegans, we take the anger, channel it, and live in a way that, to the greatest extent possible, affirms the intrinsic worth of animals. Veganism is us living in the world the way we want the world to be, and denying the violence done in our names. Equivocating on the issues and simply failing to do what is right because it is more convenient does absolutely nothing to mitigate this violence. For each egg, a chicken suffers in unusually horrible confine-ment for hours and hours; the production of milk leads to the slaughter of tens of thousands of calves for veal every year in the US alone; and just about every other animal product we can think of leads to the death or suffering of someone who is probably at least as sentient as the dog or cat that you con-sider to be a family member. Conveniently obscured from the average consumer when they buy animal flesh, eggs, or milk at the grocery store, the suffering is still there, the hidden but ever-present ingredient in every animal product. While most everyone knows somewhere in the back of their brain that animals die for their food, most people fail to acknowledge it fully at either an intellectual or emotional level. For them, the psychological distance between their cheese or eggs or steak and the real, hideous, and sorrowful lives and deaths that animals experience is hidden behind euphemisms — "meat," instead of flesh; "free range" instead of unfreedom — and cultural fairy tales about animals gamboling about in a rural paradise of verdant pastures. In this ideological cover-up that pervades our entire culture, people get to have their meat, dairy, and eggs and eat them too, all while someone else — most likely, an undocumented, under-aged, exploited worker[2] — does the dirty work to get those products to them. Animals also suffer lives of utter and total misery throughout the whole process, even in "organic," "local," "free-range," and "humane" farming operations that are supposed to be some-how better. We don't care what Whole Foods says: there is no humane animal product, period.

To be vegan is to have the guts to deny the fairy tale of the harmless animal product. To be vegan is to deny the psychological distance between the flesh in the Styrofoam tray at the supermarket and the someone — not the something — who that meat came from. To be vegan is to live fully and honestly with yourself about how animals are treated, and it is about your not taking place in that exploitative system to the greatest extent possible. Veganism is not only an affirmation about how we want the world to be, it is a lived form of protest, and our reminding people that everything is not quite right when it comes to how we treat animals. A form of everyday heroism in a world gone terribly wrong, veganism is your refusal to participate in a system that is ethically bankrupt. It is bravery in a time of cowardice.

For your refusal of this system to be sensible, it has to be complete. It cannot be something you do part time or once in a while and still have it make any ethical or logical sense. People are usually confused on this point, but think of it like this: if someone decides that breaking into people's homes is a moral wrong, and they decide that in order to decrease the impact of their crimes, they're only going to break into homes on Thursdays, are they still committing the moral wrong? The answer is obvious. While the thief may have reduced the extent of her thievery, she's still violating the law — she's just doing it less often. Similarly, if you decide that animals do not deserve to be used to produce food and clothing for you, and as a response, you eat meat only one day per week, you are still taking part in the perpetuation of a moral wrong, even if you can argue that you've reduced the extent of the harm. Reducing the consumption of animal products is nice and probably better for your health, but ultimately it isn't meaningful as a response to the problem of the injustice animals suffer unless you go all the way. The idea that less of a moral wrong is better than more of a moral wrong is kind of obvious, but as the hypothetical above shows, it misses the point badly. Without a doubt, a little animal abuse is preferable to a lot of animal abuse, but as an ethical vegan, you should be promoting a situation in which no animal abuse is taking place, and the first place you should be promoting it is in your life. Some people have accused us of being taking an absolutist position about this, claiming that the world really is made up of shades of grey, and that we should simply stop asking people to do the right thing by going vegan, and instead encourage them to reduce their consumption of animal products rather than cutting them out altogether. This kind of soft-headed logic is nice to a fault, and it misses the point of veganism almost completely. By failing to accord animals inherent moral worth — which is to say, by looking at animals solely as things that we use and control for our own interests — the idea that a little less animal abuse is sensible makes the mistake of treating animals differently than humans for no good reason. To take the example of criminality a bit farther, while we all might agree that it is generally better for a pedophile to violate two instead of three children, we can recognize that a pedophile violating any children is inherently wrong because of the harms in inflicts on the child. Similarly, were you to be kidnapped and held against your will, we would not applaud the genteel sensibilities of your kidnapper for giving you a comfortable bed to sleep in while he imprisoned you. Instead, we would decry his violation of your rights as an absolute moral wrong, and behave appropriately toward him.

It may seem inapt and even offensive to some of you to compare eating animal products to things like pedophilia and kidnapping, but the essential moral point is the same in all of the cases. In each case, a moral right is being violated — the only difference is that in the cases that involve humans, we have an easier time seeing the problem because we can identify with the subject of the comparison. Because we all have grown up in a culture that unjustly marginalizes animals as insensate brutes who will never have anything close to human worth and intelligence, it can even take those of us who have an understanding that the enslavement of animals is wrong a long time to stop applying these fuzzy and illogical moral lenses to issues. Yet, if we want to be logically and morally coherent, we have to begin working from a moral and ethical position that gets at the root of the problem, and which accords animals a set of basic, inviolable rights. (We discuss these rights and the social and cultural foundations for them in Chapter 2.) These basic rights for animals are the foundation of ethical veganism, and the only sensible way to actually combat the intersecting problems and processes that produce and reproduce the human domination of animals. Really, though, it comes down to this: if you want to abolish animal exploitation and if you truly care about animal rights, you must be vegan. There is simply no logical way that you can say you care about animals while you go on eating them or the commodities they produce.

Why Not Vegetarianism?

> *Without making any claims to self-righteousness, we feel in a strong position to criticise lacto-vegetarianism, because the worst we can say will be but a repetition of criticism we have already levelled against ourselves. Therefore we shall express the Truth as we see it and feel it, and though our friends the lacto-vegetarians may reject our ideas if they wish, we hope they will not reject us for stating them.*[3]

Even though you may agree with the ideas behind ethical veganism on a philosophical level, you may have the idea that veganism is just too far out there, too much work, and too damn annoying to deal with. As a compromise at this point, you may be either deciding to go or stay vegetarian, because, really, that just seems so much more reasonable a solution. Plus, you could never imagine giving up cheese, or cream in your coffee, or scrambled eggs, or whatever other animal product you regularly crave.

We get where you're at, but you need to move beyond this kind of thinking if you truly care about animals. While vegetarianism may be a comfortable place for you to land for animal rights reasons, vegetarianism involves habits of consumption that create conditions of extreme discomfort and death for the animals that you claim to care about. Hey, don't shoot the messenger: we spent so much time as smug, self-assured "ethical" ovo-lacto vegetarians that we understand the mindset particularly well. We thought we were doing something good with our vegetarianism, but it turns out, we were just part of the problem, and if you're a vegetarian who eats eggs and dairy and other animal products, you're part of the problem, too. Yeah, that's a bit of a blunt way to put it, but before you throw down the book and get all angry at us for being radical vegan assholes, give some consideration to these two huge reasons why vegetarianism is a poor response to the problem of animal exploitation.

HUGE REASON #1

Whereas eating meat directly involves the death of the animal to get the flesh, many vegetarians assume that consuming eggs and dairy doesn't kill any animals. Thus, the reasoning goes, eating those products is not a problem because no lives are taken. This approach is inherently flawed because it does not take into consideration the operation of modern, intensive agricultural production. The one thing that you should never forget is that animal agriculture is a globalized business that strives to maximize profits on the backs of animals and to achieve the greatest possible efficiencies. With very slim profit margins throughout the industry, producers cannot afford to waste anything, and you can bet that they will not keep animals around who are non-productive. So, first and foremost, this means that the chickens who lay eggs are inevitably slaughtered when their productivity declines beyond a certain point. The industry has insidious ways of disposing of so-called "spent hens" that range from miniature gas chambers to electrocution to neck breaking. The only thing the chickens have done to meet such ends is being unlucky enough to be born as an egg-laying hen. In a similar way, the cows who are producing milk meet their end when they fail to "yield" the right averages for the herd; this can be brought on by their age, or even by an infection or other illness. Most dairy cows who have arrived at the end of their so-called "useful" lifespan end up slaughtered many, many years before they would die naturally, after which they are rendered into ground beef and other constituent parts.

The other obvious issue that no one is ever encouraged to think about is the case of the males involved in this whole process. Egg-laying hens and dairy cows are both female. Since animals roughly tend to give birth to females and males in a 50-50 ratio, where do the approximately 50 percent of males end up? In the case of egg-laying hens, the males are absolutely worthless to the producer. If they can't lay eggs, and they're not good for meat,[4] to raise them would simply be a waste of money, and no egg producer — free range, or not, organic or not, the ones who sell to Whole Foods or not — is in this business to lose loads of money by being a farm sanctuary for hundreds or thousands non-productive (and thus, non-profitable) animals. Because of this, the unwanted, unneeded, and unprofitable animals are essentially disposable. Male chicks are often discarded at birth by being ground up alive and used for "raw protein," or they're simply thrown in dumpsters to starve and suffocate slowly — an act of unimaginable cruelty.

The male progeny of dairy cows face a similar end. Males cannot produce milk, and so are worthless for the dairy farmer, who, like the egg producer, does not want unprofitable mouths to feed around his farm.[5] Male calves, then, are usually forcibly separated from their mothers and sold at auction within days after they are born, often ending up as veal calves. Deeply confused and likely terrified by the absence of their mothers, these newborns with a herd instinct scarcely have a chance to understand the world before they are chained by the neck, all alone, inside tiny crates where they can barely move, lest their muscles grow too much. Because veal with a pinkish hue fetches the best prices at market, these horribly unfortunate animals — animals who are clearly sentient, who clearly feel and comprehend the world around them — will spend their entire short lives this way, suffering and confused, sentenced to what is demonstrably a hell on earth, all because of that supposedly "harmless" system of dairy production that provides the milk ovo-lacto vegetarians drink. As you can see, harmless eggs and harmless milk are fantasies, and if you're a vegetarian, now is the time to own up and stop living the lie. You might soothe yourself with excuses for why you cannot change, but ultimately, those excuses do nothing to help the animals that you, as a so-called "animal rights vegetarian," claim to care about.

HUGE REASON #2

The other big reason that so-called "animal rights" ovo-lacto vegetarianism is pointless has to do with the essential problem of the relationship of dominance that humans assert over animals. Veganism as a social movement — and if we're going to get serious about veganism, we have to begin building a movement that goes beyond mere consumerism — seeks to redefine the ways in which humans relate to animals. To be an ethical vegan is to demand that animals are accorded rights that cannot be violated for mere reasons of convenience, taste, or tradition. Many of the basic rights that vegans who wish to abolish animal exploitation push for are rights that would look pretty similar to the ones that we all cherish, including the right not to be the property of another, the right of bodily integrity and safety, and the right not to be used solely as the means to another's ends (we get into all of this at length in the next chapter). Put most simply, we are looking to abolish animal slavery by according animals a set of inalienable rights.

Considering all of this, even if it were somehow possible to produce dairy and eggs that did not result in the death of billions of animals a year, a producer still must confine and control animals to produce these commodities for consumers — consumers which clearly include legions of ovo-lacto vegetarians. Fully the property of another, the animals involved in these forms of production are little more to their owners than living machines for profit, slaves who day in and day out for every single day of their lives suffer solely to fulfill demands extraneous to their own desires and needs. Though the particulars of confinement and slavery may differ slightly by setting, the same basic and underlying dynamic holds whether the products in question are the typical ones in your grocery store, or whether they are labeled "cage-free," "local," "organic," or even "free-range." The myth of a compassionate animal product is just that: a myth.

As people who care about animals, we have a heavy burden to bear, one that deserves our utmost attention and our greatest effort. The enormity of the task is overwhelming, but we can all begin to make a change if we work at it together. The good news is that you are in a position to do something about it, and to make positive changes in your life that recognize the inherent worth of animals as fellow beings. The bad news is that as billions — yes, billions — of animals die each year for no good reason whatsoever, we can no longer afford self-indulgent half-measures and wishy-washy excuses that damn more and more animals to lives and deaths of total misery. Instead of looking for the path of least resistance, we have to seize control of our lives and live as examples. We have to work constantly to redefine and rethink the relationship between humans and animals, and to model changes in this relationship in our daily lives to those around us. We owe at least this much to those that we purport to care about, those who cannot speak for themselves. It comes down to this: if you care about the well being of animals, and you object to their needless suffering and death, you must stop remaking the dynamics that exploit animals in the first place. As a lived form of protest, veganism is the expression of this desire for justice, a visceral and logical reaction to the horrors visited on others in our name. It is time to give up the quaint relic that is vegetarianism, and take the first and most essential step in combating a system that treats animals not as creatures who can feel and love and think, but instead as mere engines for the production of profit. It is time to take that step and go vegan.

Just Go Vegan Already

If you're ready to stop taking part in the suffering and torture being done to animals in your name, there is only one solution: go vegan! As billions upon billions of animals are killed each year simply for reasons of taste and convenience, our plea is a somewhat urgent one. The sooner more of you out there go vegan and stay vegan, the sooner we can stem the tide of suffering — and veganism is really the only effective way to make any real change.

We get the resistance that some of you probably have at this point. Until you do it, going vegan seems like a huge, and potentially difficult change in the way you live your life, but the basics really are not that complex at all, and it is far easier than it looks. Once you make the leap, you'll wonder why you hadn't done it sooner, and if you're like us, in your quieter moments of reflection a few months out, you'll look back and feel a bit guilty for the incredibly weak excuses you had for not doing it. Bob whined for a long while about not being able to have cream in his coffee. Jenna's plaintive cries were largely for what she thought would be the end of excellent baked goods. Obviously, we now know that there are wonderful vegan substitutes for those things (which we discuss in Chapter 4), but at the time, going vegan just seemed like such a steep hill for us to climb. Since then, though, the experience of the thousands of vegans who have written to us has convinced us that the difficulties of going vegan are relatively few, at least for the most basic questions of what you decide to put in your mouth, day in and day out.

One of the reasons that going vegan can feel harder than it really is, is because we all have a tendency to baby ourselves a bit more than is probably reasonable when it comes to food and comfort. Far from being just mere nourishment, food is a complex social and cultural good whose emotional attachments are woven through our lives. Because of this, there's likely a part of all of us that is a bit irrational about our attachments to certain foods, and the emotional ties that we have to food run very deep. The example of immigrant communities shows just how far this attachment goes, and how deeply food is interwoven with our social and cultural context. When a new immigrant group arrives in a country, successive generations will often take on more and more aspects of the society into which they've immigrated. Mother-tongues often lose favor to the local language, old customs of dress may fall by the wayside, and certain customs may be discarded in favor of local habits. Even when language and dress and everything else diminish in importance for successive generations, the preferences for certain kinds of cultural dishes still hang around. This doesn't mean that someone from South Asia living in London will always on every possible occasion choose dal over chips dipped in brown sauce, but it does often mean that on special occasions, foods from the "old country" will make an appearance, and often these foods will be integral to the way a family celebrates.

For a lot of us, food is also a source of comfort. Maybe your mom's macaroni and cheese is the ultimate comfort food that can make you feel better when you're deep in the dumps, or maybe you like to eat ice cream or chocolate when you're feeling a bit low. All of us have foods that we enjoy when we're upset or sick or otherwise in need of comfort, and there's absolutely nothing wrong with that dynamic (unless you overindulge, in which case, you're probably not making the healthiest decision possible). These kinds of complex emotional attachments can help explain why otherwise rational adults will sometimes hold out on making the change to a more compassionate way of living, even when they know and logically understand the reasons for such a switch. Understanding this relationship between us and the food we eat can help you come to terms with how this might operate in your life. And to be clear, we don't want you to cut your cultural ties, starve yourself, or otherwise eat things you don't want to eat. We just want to get you to shift your comfort foods and cultural traditions to things that won't needlessly kill other beings. There's absolutely no reason that we, as vegans, cannot take our old traditions and our old favorites and rethink them as cruelty-free masterpieces that fulfill the many dimensions of food.

Still, looking at food as more than mere nourishment, it becomes a bit easier to understand the psychological and emotional barriers that many of us face when contemplating a choice that will change the way we eat, even if we recognize that the change is for the better on the whole. We are quite sympathetic to the complexity of the situation, but we believe that the complexity is best addressed by bold and decisive action that puts your potential for change at the fore, and which also minimizes the amount of time that you'll feel the separation anxiety for the foods you might be afraid of missing — and you probably won't even miss them that much anyway, to be honest.

Towards that end, our advice is simple: stop eating animal products today. Yes — today! And why not? In this world where so many of us often feel overwhelmed by social injustice and powerless to affect change, right now at this very moment, you have the chance to make a real and meaningful impact in the lives of others through your actions. In a world of insane and bloody exploitation that takes the lives of billions of animals a year, we need people with your courage — people who will stand up, be counted, and say "enough is enough." This kind of firm belief and action is the only thing that has ever really changed the world for the better, and we need you to be a part of it. It requires moral fortitude, however, because standing up for what is right isn't always easy, particularly when so many people walking around in the world see absolutely nothing wrong with drinking a glass of milk or gnawing on the dead flesh from a chicken's leg. As we said earlier, there is no doubt that you will look like the freak on occasion — but so what? If the rest of the world considers the horrendous torture and exploitation done in their names to be "normal," aren't you overvaluing normal a bit too much if you know that it is wrong, yet you cannot change because you fear looking like the freak on occasion, or because you are afraid you'll miss cream in your coffee?

Taking matters into your own hands and going vegan right now is also extraordinarily powerful — no one can do the vegan thing for you. You have to do it yourself. Only you have the power to make this change in your life, and unless you're a teenager with little control over your food purchases, you're also the only person who can stop you from doing it, too. By asserting how you want to live in the world and making today the day you come out as a vegan, you are setting a positive example for others. You're also giving yourself permission to live your life on your own terms, and that's no small personal accomplishment in a world full of teachers, professors, parents, politicians, bosses, and others who all think they know how to run your life better than you do. Truth is, they don't. Only one person truly knows how to live your life well, and that's you. If you decide that the pain and suffering inflicted in your name is wrong, now is the time to dig deep, grasp the opportunity for change, and start living your life affirmatively in a way that matches your principles.

As much as we'd like to tell you that we have an army of people ready to occupy the barricades in this particular struggle, and that you can sit back and relax because "we got this one," we can say no such thing. For veganism to work as a meaningful form of resistance, for us to make a dent in this juggernaut of animal exploitation, people like you have to step up and do the right thing. There won't magically come a time when the hard work of others will produce a sudden revolutionary break from the current system in which animals suffer horrible lives of near-total deprivation. Because of how deeply-rooted this particular form of domination is, change will take time and no small amount of commitment on the part of many of us. We can't sit around and wait for the revolution that frees the animals we claim to care about. Instead, we have to be that revolution, living it in our lives and feeling it in our hearts. It is in our spirit, or it is nowhere.[6] Together, we all will be the ones who will chart a course for a non-violent post-exploitative world, and our veganism can give others a glimpse of what this world could look like. We can only make this world happen by living it as the best vegans we can be, day in and day out.

The thing is, time is wasting as billions of animals are slaughtered each year. The consumption of animal products continues to grow, and even well-meaning people who should know better are now copping out by eating supposedly "compassionate" or "humane" local meats that have since become profitable niches for retailers everywhere. Never has the time been more urgent. We need to get going, and we need to get going now. That's why you have to make the commitment to go vegan today — not tomorrow, not next week, and not once you've eaten the eggs out of your fridge. We need you in the struggle now. We really can't wait much longer.

The Cold Tofu Approach

Our approach to getting you to go vegan takes into consideration the necessity of immediacy while also bearing in mind the powerful emotional connections that food can have. If you are willing to throw yourself into it and not cheat, this approach works. It has worked repeatedly for many people the world over, and it worked for us. It will probably also work for you, too, if you make an agreement with yourself to take it seriously.

Our approach begins with a challenge. Many claim to care deeply for animals, and we have frequently heard people say that there isn't anything they wouldn't do to help stop the suffering animals experience. Our guess is that if you picked up this book, you are one of these people who cares enough about animals to at least contemplate giving up eating them and their products, and that care is commendable in world like ours that is full of people who can't be bothered to care about much of anything. But let's see you put your money where your mouth is. If you truly do care, you should care enough not to eat animals, and today is the day that you should make a pledge that you will go vegan for at least the next 21 days. This isn't that much to ask, really. We're not expecting you to ride across the country on a bike without a seat, or looking for your permission to slide bamboo slivers under your fingernails. We're just asking that you ante up, make your commitment real, and not eat any animal products at all for three weeks. Three weeks is nothing! Surely, you can persist; people with less spine than you have been vegan for decades.

In order to make this work, however, there are two things you must do: you must quit all animal products cold tofu, and you must educate yourself about veganism. Neither is optional if you want to be successful, so read on about how to make a clean break from your life of consuming cruelty.

1. YOU HAVE TO QUIT ANIMAL PRODUCTS COLD TOFU — AND NO CHEATING!

This means no dairy, no eggs, no meat, no fish, no honey, and no other animal byproducts — not even a little! In the subsequent chapters, we tell you all that you need to know to effectively do this, so don't sweat it if you're not sure exactly what it is that you'll need to be avoiding in terms of hidden ingredients and the like — you're holding the book in your hands that will walk you through all of it carefully, just read on. The important thing right at this moment is making the commitment, and your getting a sense during the coming weeks of what it is like to be a vegan.

We are insistent about your not cheating not because we believe in total purity for the sake of purity itself, but because we're trying to get you to overcome your ties to the old foods that you love but which are also caught up in circuits of animal exploitation. If you are trying to get away from these foods, and you give in and let yourself have some, you're only going to want more. Slowly and insidiously, the food that you're trying to give up will only gain more power over you as you begin to look forward to that tiny, little bite each day, or however often you end up convincing yourself that it is justifiable to indulge. It just becomes way too easy to fall back into old habits if you don't step away from the animal products you're trying to give up. Before too long, that innocent enough feeling of "Well, it won't really matter if I have just one tiny bite" becomes "Well, I already had one bite, so what's a few more?" which, in time, becomes "Fuck it. I've already gone this far, might as well go all the way and just eat as much as I want." Then, next thing you know, you're off ordering three-cheese pizzas like some stoned alt-bro[7] maxing out mommy's credit card. To our way of thinking, it is easier just to put up with the annoyance of not having a food you like for a week or two, after which you will probably find your desire for it waning drastically, since it only takes a few weeks for your tastes to change anyway.

Though not cheating is easy for a lot of foods, some people find giving up cheese particularly difficult. For us, it wasn't hard. We just went vegan one day, and didn't look back, but for a lot of people we've talked to, cheese is the lone item that often still has its hooks in them. So many people have complained to us about how hard it was to give up cheese that we almost felt like we needed to set up some kind of support group in the basement of an area church where we served burnt coffee (with soy creamer) and let people talk about how many days cheese-clean they've been. Frankly, the whole thing was perplexing for us until we read up on casomorphins, or opioid chemicals that are present in cow's milk (and by extension, very much present in cheese). Evolutionarily, these peptides probably had the function of creating a positive association between the calf and its mother and her milk. Now, however, humans consume more cow's milk than calves do, and — improbable though it sounds — those who consume large amounts of dairy products are probably mildly addicted to them. It isn't like you're going to get the DTs or have seizures if you give up cheese, but certainly, if they operate as some theorize, these opiate effects can help to explain the more than mild cravings that lots of people have. A study underway during the time we were writing this book is looking at how casomorphins work in the human body, operating under the functional hypothesis that because cheese is one of the most commonly craved foods, it may be exerting mild opiate effects on its consumers.[8] If this hypothesis is true the correct solution isn't weaning yourself from ~~crack~~cheese slowly. As we suggest above, that would probably only lead you back to eating more cheese. The right solution is to stop eating cheese now, and to make an agreement with yourself never to eat it again. If you feel tempted to eat it, slide a paperclip over this page, and when you're on the verge of eating cheese, come back here and remind yourself of these disgusting cheese facts:

> Cheese is made from milk, and milk almost always contains at least some pus. You may comfort yourself by thinking that the pus is pasteurized, and certainly, pasteurization will prevent you from becoming ill, but you're still eating pus. Look at it like this: you could stick a dog turd in an autoclave and render it biologically harmless with significant pressure and heat. Yet, we're willing to wager that you'd not be anxious to eat it unless you have some very strange proclivities indeed.

> Forget about being vegan — most cheeses aren't even vegetarian. Rennet, a stomach enzyme common to most mammals, is used to make cheese by "digesting" it, leaving behind a solid and a liquid. Rennet is often harvested from the stomachs of cattle in slaughterhouses, and used directly in cheese. Though there are vegetarian rennets synthesized by other means, it is difficult to know which cheeses use vegetarian rennet and which cheeses use the stuff scraped out of the stomachs of slaughtered animals. Yum! Cow stomach excretions obviously go great with pus!

> In order for you to have your beloved cheese, someone had to produce the milk to make the cheese, and we don't mean a dairy farmer. The someone in this case is a nameless dairy cow, identified only by a number and probably an radio frequency identification tag in her ear that helps the ~~slave owner~~ farmer track her productivity so he can send her to slaughter once she underproduces. In the larger dairy operations, this cow may never go outside, and she will repeatedly give birth to calves who will be

stolen from her almost immediately after they are born. She will live a short and miserable life, and end up as hamburger on the plate of some fast food consumer, all because you could not find the guts up to stop eating cheese or drinking milk. And you say you care about animals?

> Beyond being a disaster for cows, cheese is a disaster for you. A cup of diced cheddar has a whopping 532 calories, 385 of which come from fat. That includes 28 grams of saturated fat, which is 139 percent of amount recommended for total daily consumption by the United States government. To all that fat, you can add 139 milligrams of cholesterol and 820 mg of sodium. For comparison, if you decided to reach for a cup of chopped carrots instead, you'd be taking in fewer than a tenth of the total calories (52 calories for the whole cup) and less than 1 percent of the fat (3 calories versus 385 calories) than if you ate the cheese.[9]

Cheese may taste good to you now, but really, like every other animal product, there's no good reason to eat it. It is bad for you and bad for the animals that have to make the raw ingredients that go into it. Give it up now, call it quits, and go cold tofu. If you can do that, maybe you can come to our cheese-eaters anonymous meetings, sip some bad coffee, and tell us how many days you've been clean.

Though we focus on cheese because in our experience it tends to be the most difficult thing for people to give up, there are no doubt those of you out there reading now who have different foods that you are worried about parting ways with. Whatever it may be, the advice is the same: just stop eating it, and don't go back to eating it. Be strong about it, use your willpower, and remember why you're doing this in the first place. Don't allow yourself to fall prey to those internal monologues in which you feel badly for yourself, or appeal to your inner child. Instead, if you want to cheat, think about the animal that had to suffer and probably die to produce that product. If you have a dog or a cat or another animal who is part of your family, think about how it would feel if you knew that your beloved family member were in that situation, or if you yourself were. This is the first and most essential step of any form of compassion, the ability to put yourself in the position of another who suffers. Indeed, this is one of the most prominent gifts endowed upon humanity, so use it for the betterment of others. Remember that for eggs, chickens are often crammed six or seven deep into a space the size of an office filing cabinet drawer for their entire lives. For dairy, calves must be separated from their mothers, and they are often killed at a very young age. For meat, throats must be slit, and blood must be drained. For fish, sea animals must spend their final minutes painfully gasping for oxygen that will never come. Anyone who is not a sociopath would not wish these kinds of horrific ends on anyone. And while lots of self-interested businesses with money to make from their exploitation of animals may try to tell you that the eggs are gathered humanely, or that the animals are sung a mellifluous song before the bolt action of the stunner punctures the white matter of their brain in a final moment of confusion and terror, they're all deeply full of shit, because they all have something to gain by getting you to believe these myths about "humane" products that could never, ever possibly be anything even remotely approaching humane. It doesn't matter which main-stream animal rights group has told you so, or endorsed the store or the farm. We'll say it again, in case it isn't sinking in: there are simply no humane animal products, period.

On the issue of self-interest, you probably think you could say the same about us and veganism: that if we can convince you to go vegan, we gain, and so we're not a disinterested party either. Well, fair enough. We will readily admit to you that we are not disinterested. We want to see an end to this ridiculous and unnecessary bloodbath, and we want to convince you to dig deep and find the heroism in your heart to be part of the fight against it too. But when all is said and done, we have nothing much to gain on a personal level if you go vegan. You probably already bought the book if you're this far in; at this point, our meager royalty has already been paid to us. Whole Foods, however — they want you to eat their Compassion Certified beef and free-range eggs for life. Same with the local grass-fed, free-range guy in your area, the very mention of whom, we are sure, would bring a small rush of blood to Michael Pollan's withered, omnivorous nether-regions. Always remember that animal exploiters exploit animals not for some higher good of "feeding people," but instead to make a profit from their exploitation. As more and more consumers show ambivalence about the violence done to animals, the producers have to convince you that they care in order to keep you buying the products of suffering they produce. To do that, they will go to any reasonable end possible, because they know that this is something that hits at the heart of their business.

Point is, if you find yourself ready to chow down on some random animal product, you have to remind yourself that someone out there had to be confined, suffer, and die to make that product, just so you can feel a little better for having eaten it, all while perfectly suitable and healthy plant-based alternatives surround you. If you can imagine the ways in which your consumption is linked to these forms and circuits of production, you can begin to evolve a compassionate approach to your life, which in turn will help you to resist animal products during the first few weeks when they seem the most tempting. If you can stick with this for three weeks, though, and you keep reminding yourself of the inherent cruelty involved in animal products, there's every chance that your cravings will be replaced by revulsion, and you will be a vegan for life — which is obviously the only way to be if you're ready to stand up and say "iya basta!" or "enough is enough!" when it comes to the ways in which we abuse animals.

2. **YOU MUST ACTIVELY EDUCATE YOURSELF DURING THESE 21 DAYS.**

In this book, we take it as our job to help you learn the most you can about veganism in a single book that won't break the bank or wear you out with excessive detail. In the coming chapters, you'll learn about the philosophical and theoretical foundations of the abolitionist approach to animal rights, how to avoid hidden ingredients in all manner of things, how to deal with social situations as a vegan, and lots of other useful information that will get you moving in the right direction towards being a happy and lifelong vegan. While we aim to be as complete a resource as we can be for you, one of the important things that we cannot teach you is how to cook. No worries, though: plenty of other vegans have written amazing vegan cookbooks that cover just about every conceivable cuisine, cooking for every possible occasion, and ideas for meals that range from the simple and quick to the complex and gourmet — the variety will amaze you. Add to this selection of fine cookbooks an ever-expanding vegan cooking blogosphere spilling over with pictures, ideas, and recipes, and a huge website loaded with user-submitted recipes like vegweb.com, and you will never be at a loss for vegan things to cook.

As you're getting going in your veganism, make sure to consult a few of the resources we recommend in Chapter 4 so that you can begin to learn the ins-and-outs of vegan cookery. For those of you that already like to cook, this can be an amazing time to discover the new repertoire of foods and techniques that go along with vegan cooking. You can use this opportunity not only to eat new foods that you rarely or never ate as a vegetarian or omnivore, but also to dig into new cuisines whose traditional cooking styles are well-suited to a plant-based diet. Conversely, if you aren't really into cooking, fear not. You don't need to love to cook to be a healthy and happy vegan, but you, too, should take the time to learn how to prepare at least a few easy things that you enjoy and which are also healthful. As you'll read later, we believe that self-sufficiency is important to being a successful vegan, so learning to cook some basic dishes that you can expand upon later is really not a bad idea, so that you don't have to rely on others to provide vegan food for you. This is easier than it sounds, and there are cookbooks that have lots of delicious but easy recipes that you can try out. We can accept that some of you may never learn to love cooking, but if you can get yourself to look at it as something other than a chore, you may find yourself getting more interested in it, because now your cooking means more than just nourishment: it is just another expression of your living your life well as a vegan. A little time invested here will pay off for you in the long run.

While you are checking out the cookbooks and cooking websites we recommend, start planning out the menus for a few meals, go shopping, and pick up the ingredients so that you're not at a loss for what to eat. The advanced planning may seem like a pain if you're used to winging it, but it can be really useful, especially at first.[10] If you happen to arrive home after a busy day at work and you didn't have time to go to the store, you might find yourself staring at an empty fridge and thinking about ordering some takeout whose veganness you find yourself unsure of because you're a bit overwhelmed by what to make, and feeling a bit lazy on top of it all. Though this sounds like some trite mantra from some overpaid life coach, one of the biggest keys to success in just about anything is putting yourself in a situation where you can be successful. Having food in the house and a game plan for a few meals that you can cook on the spot will help you to find success easily when it comes to getting started down your path to veganism. Showing up at home exhausted after a long day of work and trying to sort out a new way of eating without the right foods in your house or an idea of how to cook them is just setting yourself up for making the wrong choices. We'll state advice here on living well as a vegan that you're going to see throughout this book in various forms: namely, when possible, you can save yourself a lot of trouble as a vegan by simply planning ahead.

If you're like Bob, planning ahead is something for organized people without ADHD, so it may strike you as incredibly dull. Still, there's a lot to be said for it, and for looking at this planning as part of what you have to do to throw yourself into veganism with the most enthusiasm possible. Whatever you do, don't let yourself get bogged down early on over what you cannot (or really, to be more accurate, will not) eat. Too many people look at this period in their new vegan lives as a kind of mourning period for the animal foods that are no longer part of their diets. Emotions like these are understandable, but you should try to cultivate a new kind of consciousness about this choice you've made. Focusing on the negatives of veganism and all the things that you "cannot" have will only make you feel deprived, and this is a new and exciting time in your life, a time that you've decided to take a personal yet public stand, and to live in a way that's consistent with your values. Being the human that you are, you could choose to exercise the privilege that comes to you through your species and eat dairy, eggs, flesh, and fish, but you instead choose not to because you know that avoiding these things is the choice that sides with the just and the right. Having made your stance on the side of justice, you should stay firmly there, and recognize that there is something personally and socially powerful in that stance — you're remaking the world in a powerful way with your choices and actions. If you start to feel like you're backsliding into exasperation, remind yourself of the positive commitment that you are making by going vegan and staying vegan, and realize that from this day forward, you are part of the struggle to gain social justice for animals.

Apart from fretting over missed foods, there's another issue when it comes to food and eating that is worth mentioning. Too many of us — omnivore, vegetarian, and vegan alike — devote too little time, money, and effort to the food that we consume. As a result, many of us are also malnourished. We're going to sound like giant, crystal-clutching hippies here, but in all seriousness, the malnourishment is nutritional as well as personal. Food can connect us to other people, and sharing food is often at the center of making happy memories. Cooking and eating together is a fantastic way of strengthening interpersonal and family bonds, whether those bonds are between children and parents, spouses, friends, or even between humans and their companion animals.[11] Plus, when you prepare your own food, you know what is in it, and you can gain a deep sense of satisfaction from having made something delicious. And on another level altogether, food provides the fuel for us to survive. Though most of us don't often think about it, our bodies are remaking themselves during every single moment of our existence, sloughing off old cells and excreting waste, while simultaneously building everything back up. As a result, food has a central and intimate role in the lives of each and every one of us as the primary resource fueling this remarkable process of regeneration. Like the old adage suggests, we actually are made up of what we eat. Considering that, are you going to give your body and mind the foods that it needs to function at optimal efficiency — foods like greens, grains, beans, and fresh vegetables — or are you going to slow it down with processed crap laden with preservatives whose names you cannot even begin to pronounce?

A healthy attitude about food and cooking is vitally important not only to the long-term success of your veganism, but also to your own long-term well being. Devoting a little time and potentially some expense to watching out for this essential aspect of your veganism will pay off in the long run, as you'll have a wider repertoire of foods to choose from, and you'll have a sense of how to prepare them. By giving your diet a bit more thought and some of the time it rightly deserves, you can ensure that you are eating a wide variety of foods, which is essential to your mental and physical health (vegan or not, variety in one's diet is always a good thing). And finally, whatever you do in these first few weeks, don't fall into the dangerous trap of relying solely on processed foods like veggie burgers, french fries, fake lunchmeats and sausages, and veganized sweets. These things are now pretty easy to get at most grocery stores in North America and Europe, and while eating these foods occasionally is probably not detrimental to your health in the long run, you will probably end up sick if your diet is too heavy with this stuff. If you're in this for the reasons we are — to stop the exploitation of animals — you need to be as healthy as you can be, not only to serve as an example to others about how vegans can be healthy and happy, but also to help us fight this fight with your own activism. The temptation is always there to take the easy way out and eat the processed shit, but you should try to remind yourself that no one — not you, not the vegan movement, and not the animals — benefits from you getting sick because you are not eating enough of a variety of foods, or because you haven't taken your vitamin B12. (We cover these points in more depth in Chapter 4.)

One final point on the topic of food: some of you may be worrying that vegan food is too expensive to be a realistic option for you. While it is undeniably true that there are expensive vegan specialty products, you do not have to eat any of them to be a happy and healthy vegan. If you stay away from fake meats, fake cheeses, processed foods, frozen entrees, and the like, you can actually buy plenty of healthy vegan food without breaking the bank. Though we give you more advice about this in Chapter 4, a quick example might help to drive home the point. In the United States, a company called Amy's Kitchen makes a frozen roasted vegetable vegan pizza that is widely available. (To give you a sense of just how widely available, we could even get these in the remote and desolate rural wasteland we lived in while writing most of this book.) Perhaps we're just exceptionally hungry vegans, but a single pizza from Amy's is not really even enough for the two of us to split for lunch, yet these things cost more than $9 each at our local co-op. For that same $9, we can make a huge batch of hummus, and buy enough tomatoes, lettuce, onions, and tortillas to eat wraps for lunch for about five days and still have money left over. Or, if you really wanted pizza, you could make and freeze several pizzas yourself for the same price as a single Amy's pizza. The point should be obvious: you can blow your cash on expensive, pre-prepared specialty foods that might carry you through one meal (if that), or you can plan ahead, think it through, and use the exact same amount of money to eat fresher, tastier food for a couple of days.

Humans do not live by food alone, so as you're sorting out the food options, make sure you also find some vegan company during these initial weeks of your veganism. If you happen a reader who lives in a city and who is already surrounded by vegans and has a clutch of vegan friends, then count yourself among the lucky. For most of the rest of you, you may be the only vegan you know, and at times, it can get lonely, if only because the world is a pretty screwed up place. As you start to get more into your veganism, things that do not bother non-vegans — say, trying to eat dinner with someone eating a dozen chicken wings as an appetizer — will probably begin to unnerve you as you start to connect the something of the chicken wing to the someone who was once a living being pecking about on the ground not all that long ago. To be blunt, these kinds of realizations can fuck with your head, and sometimes, you just need to vent to someone who will get it. Worry not! In the past several years, the Internet has become an important place for vegans and animal rights activists to connect with one another, and as a beginning vegan, you can find a comfortable spot for yourself in cyberspace. In order to facilitate some of this kind of interaction, we've set up a few outposts on the Internet that have become fairly popular over the past few years, often to our great surprise. Our forums at http://forums.veganfreak.com bring together a diverse community of users from all over the world who are serious about veganism and abolishing animal exploitation. On the forums, users find friendship, exchange and develop ideas about vegan activism, outreach, and education, share frustrations and joys, have discussions and debates, and organize local meet-ups where you can get to know lots of vegans IRL (in real life). From the outside, saying that you've met some of your best friends online is probably only a hair less geeky than saying that you are the primary author of the Boba Fett page over on Wookiepedia, but the sad truth of the matter is that we vegans tend to be few and far between, so there's nothing wrong with finding some community virtually.[12] For a large portion of the time we lived in rural, upstate New York, we were the only vegans we knew in person, an experience many of you are likely familiar with. It wasn't until we actually got a few people we knew to go vegan that we were able to have vegan friends we could see on a regular basis.

In addition to the forums, you may also want to give our podcast, *Vegan Freak Radio*, a listen. The twenty most recent episodes of the show are always available for free at http://veganfreakradio.com, so during these first few weeks as a vegan, pop by the site, and download a few shows to see what it's all about. We started this online radio show just after publishing the first edition of this book, and we've been going strong for a few years now, thanks to the enthusiasm and support of thousands of listeners from all over the world. We work hard to put out a show with professional-quality audio production, and we keep the shows lively and entertaining while also giving due attention to serious issues. On the show, we've been fortunate enough to interview a diversity of guests who are prominent in the animal rights movement, ranging from major animal rights theorists such as Professor Gary Francione (about whom you'll read more in the next chapter) to Chris Hannah from the hardcore band Propagandhi. In addition to interviews, we discuss recent news items, and take listener comments and questions via email, voicemail, and Twitter.[13] While we always produce the show with an eye towards entertainment, we primarily do the show to provide a sort of conversational hour or two of vegan company for our listeners. In the years we've been broadcasting, many people have written to tell us that they find our program to be a source of vegan companionship that they otherwise lack in their personal lives. For others who don't really need the community, it is simply an entertaining romp through current vegan issues and ideas.

Shameless self-promotion aside, we suggest that you find community not as a way of pimping the things we do to provide that community, but rather to encourage you to find connections with other vegans. In the work that we do, getting people to go vegan and stay vegan is what is most important to us, and we've found over the years of doing this that having a comfortable place to be yourself can make a huge difference.

Whether you manage to find support, friendship, and entertainment through one of our little outposts in cyberspace or whether you happen to find what you need elsewhere, the important part is that you find some place that you can feel at home, whether it is virtual or physical.

Finally, we have one last thing that you absolutely must do during your first few weeks as a vegan. Though living as a vegan can a healthful choice that is positively correlated with all kinds of beneficial health outcomes,[14] you should take the time to educate yourself about your own nutritional requirements, either by referring to the book *Becoming Vegan* by Brenda Davis and Vesanto Melina or consulting a vegan-friendly nutritionist in your area. While this is advice that all of our readers should take to heart, talking with a health care professional about your dietary needs is especially important for any of you who have any medical conditions that have specific dietary requirements. Though it depends on the condition, you may be pleasantly surprised to discover that veganism may help to alleviate problems you may be having. To take just one example, adult-onset diabetics (Type 2) are often told to eat a "low carb" diet, which most people assume automatically makes veganism impossible. Yet, Type 2 diabetics can significantly benefit from eating a low-fat, high-fiber vegan diet according to recent peer-reviewed research by Dr. Neal Barnard.[16] Point is, if you have extraordinary needs or an ongoing disorder or illness, find out what you should be eating, and devise a plan in consultation with a healthcare professional. While there is nothing inherently difficult or unhealthy about veganism that should give you pause, you are better to be on the safe side and have a full understanding of which foods can provide you with the extra or different nutrients that you need if you have a preexisting medical condition.

For the rest of you, there's not much to worry about (and we cover most of the rest of what you need to know in Chapter 4). Veganism doesn't require attention to combining particular proteins and carbs, or any other mythical nutritional hooey that you may have heard floating around out there. As long as you don't eat too many cupcakes or other junk foods, being vegan is easy and can be healthful. We've been vegan for years, and not once has either of us ended up in the doctor's office with a case of protein deficiency, or whatever other horrors people imagine befall vegans. For most of you who are already healthy, you'll usually do just fine by eating a wide variety of foods like fresh vegetables, fruits, whole grains, legumes, and natural oils like the ones found in nuts, olives, and avocados. Add to this a regular vegan multivitamin that contains B12, and you're well on the way to being a healthy vegan. (For those of you who are very active, either through the work you do, or through athletics, it is pretty much the same, but you'll just be eating more of everything.) Once you get used to being a vegan, you probably won't have to think about nutrition much at all, and you may even naturally find yourself eating more healthfully and feeling better both physically and mentally than when you were an omnivore or vegetarian.

THESE FIRST THREE WEEKS OF YOUR VEGANISM are a precious time in your life, a vibrant and exciting time that you should be enjoying and living to the fullest. Rarely do any of us get the chance to remake our lives with such an important transformation, yet by deciding to go vegan, you are committing to living in the world in a completely new way, and that's extraordinarily powerful. You're still you, and you haven't joined a cult or anything, but looking back at our first few weeks as vegans, we remember feeling almost jubilant about it. For us, going vegan felt like a big step, but it felt like the right step, because we knew it was the right thing to do despite the initial minor frustrations (and we didn't have a book like this one to help us out). We completely get that you may feel like you're on the verge of jumping from one side of a canyon to another as you make this big change in your life. There's absolutely nothing wrong with this feeling. It is natural, and even healthy, because it means that you're thinking. The gap looks big, but trust us: it isn't. As with any big leap, it takes a bit of courage to make a change, and you have to have enough of a belief in yourself to do it, and do it well. We have every bit of faith that you can do it, and you need to have that same belief in yourself to do what's obviously right.

What Veganism Isn't

You might be ready to take the leap into veganism, but we want to make sure that you're doing it for the right reasons. To be clear, we don't envision ourselves as the vegan cops, the final arbiters of what is and is not vegan, or anything like that. Instead, we're just two people who have helped a lot of others to go vegan, and along the way, we've met some vegans and ex-vegans who seem to have gone vegan for what seem to us like dubious reasons. From the outside, you might wonder why we care. You'd probably figure that we just want fewer people to be eating animals and not really care otherwise why they are or are not eating them. While we obviously want lots of people to go vegan, the reason people are vegan is important to us, because our ideas and our actions based on those ideas have to be coherent if we're going to ever make any progress. On top of this, when people aren't vegan for the right reasons, they often make for poor vegans, and end up eating non-vegan foods, which confuses everyone else about what veganism is about. At the very least, we need to have vegans who are clear exemplars of the concept, not cheese-eaters who are masquerading as vegans.

As a lived set of principles that are guided by a moral and ethical stance about the problematic relationship between humans and animals, veganism is an outright rejection of the violent and hierarchical processes that condemn animals to lives of subjugation, servitude, and oppression. Yet, many people try to turn veganism into something that it isn't, and here are a few of the things that veganism definitely is not.

IT ISN'T ABOUT YOU.

Despite popular belief, veganism isn't about you. Sure, it is about what you eat and wear and how you live, but it isn't only something that you do for yourself. As we said earlier, it is okay to feel good about being vegan: it is a positive statement and an affirmative commitment about how you're living your life. That's always refreshing and empowering, and hell yeah, you have every right to feel good about that. Plus, doing what is right always feels good, so there's some intrinsic pleasure there, too. It is okay to pat yourself on the back, and to feel a bit charged up and excited about living well and living life on your own terms. That's totally cool. The problem, though, comes when people think of veganism as some kind of inhuman, god-like sacrifice they're making on behalf of the animals. Publicly playing the martyr who has so valiantly sacrificed the so-called "dietary pleasures" cheese, dairy, eggs, and all the rest just makes you look like a self-centered asshole — plus, you become a real downer to be around. Come down off the cross, already, and stop feeling badly for yourself. All of the whinging and whining and pining for animal products and your extended soliloquies about what a fantastic martyr you are makes veganism look hard — which it isn't in the vast and overwhelming majority of cases. No one — not omnivores and especially not your fellow vegans — wants to hear the cries of a vegan who's jonesin' for a cheese fix. Muffle the cries of your extended lamentation at the loss of ice cream as a dietary staple, and hold back your whines about how wonderful a person you are for giving it up. Of course, when you first go vegan, you might miss these things, but there are excellent substitutes, and they're getting better every day (we go into a bit of depth on this in Chapter 4). Besides being viewed as an intolerable pain in the ass, you personally make real all of the omnivorous fantasies about how we're actually all just depriving ourselves of things that we really want to eat anyway because we're all horrendous food Nazis who hate pleasure. At worst, you'll lead people to believe that you're secretly sneaking these products, and they'll doubt your sincerity as a vegan, which can really make life harder for you (and for the rest of us, too). At best, people will just tire of you and tune you out. Neither end is a desirable one.

Perhaps an analogy will be useful. For example, we live all live in sexist societies — societies that value the contributions, rights, and ideas of men over those of women. If you're a man in one of these societies, you surely have a lot to gain by being a sexist and upholding these conditions of masculinity. A quick but powerful example of this is in wage disparity. In the United States, men routinely make something like 25 percent more than women performing the same job, even when every other measure is held equal. It is as though employers have collectively decided that being in possession of a set of ovaries somehow makes the reduced remuneration you receive for your labor power justifiable. Obviously, this is patently unjust, but if you're a male, you have a clear interest in upholding sexism: it literally pays! Despite this fact, many men who consider themselves allies with women's struggles for equity stand up against this and other aspects of sexism. They stand up and fight for equity because they know that sexism is wrong, and many men know that even if they can gain from it, that gain is not representative of the kind of world that they'd want to live in. Similarly, if you're an ethical vegan, you know you can personally gain a great deal by just accepting animal exploitation as "the way it has always been" and going with the path of least resistance. You can eat your [insert desired product of animal torture here] if you can just ignore the fact that animals must die to produce it. In the same way that many men comfortably uphold sexism, many meat-eaters make this very decision to accept animal suffering for taste, tradition, and convenience. It might be that both the meat-eater and the sexist imagine that things will never change, or they simply accept that this is the "natural" way of the world. In either case, they're wrong. Things can change, and you can be an agent of that change. You can be a feminist to fight sexism, and you can be a vegan to fight speciesism. As an ethical vegan, you surely know that just accepting the completely disgusting conditions of animal agriculture is wrong. The death, dismemberment, and suffering done in the name of the average meat-eating palate are a disaster on so many levels. Knowing this, you've decided to do something about it by changing yourself so you can help to create the kind of world you want to live in. In short, you're doing what's ethically and morally right.

Because of this, it is unhelpful to view veganism as some kind of heroic sacrifice on your part. Sure, you are sacrificing what you could have, just as the anti-sexist sacrifices what he could have by being opposed to sexism. But you don't really deserve the martyr points for doing what you know is right already and living by your ethics. Ethical veganism isn't exactly a sacrifice: it is more like what you must do if you want to live your life in a way that is true to your principles. If this is something you're deciding to do for principled reasons — and we think this is the only reason to go vegan — do it well, live it affirmatively and live it positively. You don't gain vegan cool points for playing the messiah, and after a while, people will just start rolling their eyes at how ridiculously Emo you are.

IT ISN'T THE PARIS EXCEPTION

"If you don't stick to your values when they're tested, they're not values. They're hobbies."

— Jon Stewart, The Daily Show, Jan. 22, 2009

Ethical veganism is the expression of a set of moral and ethical principles; it is living life consciously as an anti-speciesist. If you buy the moral and ethical antecedents of veganism — namely, that there is no compelling reason to make animals suffer for our ends[15] — it follows logically that being on vacation is not a logically and morally consistent reason to give up on your veganism. Yet, even Peter Singer — a figure who many hastily regard as the "father" of the modern animal rights movement — has said that veganism need not be adhered to strictly. In *The Way We Eat*, a book Singer co-authored with Jim Mason, Singer argued for what he called the "Paris Exception," or the notion that when one is traveling, one need not be so strict with one's veganism. Boiled down to its most essential nugget of idiocy, the Paris Exception goes something like this: if you're a tourist in Paris, don't sweat the veganism. In an interview in the now-defunct Satya magazine, Singer responds to a question about the Paris Exception, saying "...when I'm traveling and it's hard to get vegan food in some places or whatever, I'll be vegetarian." While it is probably true that there are places in the world where it is difficult to be vegan, it isn't impossible in the vast majority of situations, and usually, with a little creativity, wit, humor, and openness, you can be accommodated as a vegan if you simply go to the trouble of asking nicely.[17] Singer continues on with his absurdities: "I won't eat eggs if they're not free-range, but if they're free-range, I will. I won't order a dish that is full of cheese, but I won't worry about, say, whether an Indian vegetable curry was cooked with ghee."

To us, if you eat eggs (free range or not), you simply are not living by the principles of ethical veganism — and hence, you're not a vegan. Moreover, asking an Indian restaurant to cook your dish without ghee is trivial, and we know because we have done it many times in several countries. The danger in what Singer does here is to give people an out that we find unacceptable: if veganism is too hard, or too inconvenient, Singer essentially says, "don't sweat it, just eat the free range stuff." The problem is that the free range stuff isn't really all that much better in the long run. Animals are still killed when they're done being productive enough for producers, and you can bet that most free-range egg hatcheries (much like their non-free-range counterparts) also discard male chicks by grinding them up alive or otherwise "disposing" of them. Free range is largely a figment of marketing geniuses, designed to take your eye off of the fact that any animal agriculture violates the basic rights of animals by treating them as property and commodities.[18] Plus, how can you say that using animals for human ends is wrong if you're willing to go and use them yourself?

No doubt, some of you are getting ready to run to your email so you can send us indignant missives about how intolerant we are, and how we're being too hard on poor Professor Singer. After all, as people have said to us in the past, he has written *Animal Liberation*, and deserves some credit for that, right? The problem we see with what Singer says is this: if you can sacrifice a principled position because you don't wish to inconvenience yourself, it is worth wondering what that principle meant to you in the first place. Being an anti-speciesist is not a part-time job, and being on vacation does not absolve you of your duty to do what's right. Plus, in our experience, you learn the most about yourself and your values when they're tested in less than optimal situations, when the execution of actions based on larger principles is fraught by real-life difficulties. Really, Singer and those who tend to agree with him on this point are spilling a lot of ink for no reason. The solution is simple: if you're a vegan, be a vegan. Don't look for excuses, don't eat free range, and don't equivocate. Stop fucking around, and just be vegan.

IT ISN'T ABOUT TOTAL PURITY

We live in a world where animal exploitation is not only the norm, but also an immensely profitable set of interlocking industries. One of the ways that slaughterhouses remain profitable is to use as much of the animal as possible, including parts that most people would never imagine had any use. Bone and cartilage are rendered into products like gelatin (can you say Jell-O?) and into products that are used in industrial processes, including binding agents for tires, industrial glues, and the like. Because these uses are pervasive and often not directly documented, it is probably impossible for anyone to live fully, completely, and totally vegan. If you drive or ride a bike, your tires probably contain some slaughterhouse by-products. Similarly, if you take pharmaceuticals or other medicines, those medicines have certainly been tested on animals. Plus, harvesting grains probably kills a small number of animals as well. Despite all of this, we'd not advise that you not drive or ride your bike (you probably need to work or at least get places), we'd not suggest that you avoid taking essential medicines, and we'd certainly not suggest that you stop eating. Let's be clear: unlike Professor Singer, we believe it is reasonable and easy to give up meat, dairy, eggs, honey and other consumable animal products. It is also a simple matter to give up new purchases of leather and wool and other animal-derived products, a point that we explore in much more depth in Chapter 5. When it comes down to it, we simply don't need any of those things to live healthfully or happily, and the only reasons that people continue to eat or use them are convenience, tradition, preference, and taste. The person vacationing in Paris can avoid eggs and cheese, and so she should if she's an ethical vegan, despite what Singer says. Sure, it might be a pain, and it might mean going to an accommodating restaurant, but so what? The inconvenience is minor in the scheme of things, and if we vegans profess to care about animals, this should not be a big deal to us. Yet, let's say the same person vacationing in Paris finds herself coming down with a nasty bacterial infection after being violently attacked by a roaming flock of free-range chickens, hell-bent on revenge. Can we reasonably expect the vacationer to avoid antibiotics that could save her life because they were tested on animals, or because there's some gelatin in the capsule? Absolutely not, because in this situation, she has absolutely no other choice if she needs to live. Thus, the distinction between Singer's position and our position hinges on the notion of necessity. No one needs to eat eggs and cheese when they're on vacation in Paris, but if you get an infection that's severe enough, you obviously have no choice but to take antibiotics, or suffer the potentially deadly consequences, even if those antibiotics contain animal products, or were tested on animals.

In thinking about this, it is important to remember that the ubiquity of animal products in unavoidable places is a by-product of speciesism. We live in a world in which the social and economic systems that mediate our existence provide us with no other real alternatives to these products, some of which are absolutely essential to our health or livelihoods. In this case, because we have no real, viable alternative, we have no choice but to consume the things that we need to live. As a result, it is often difficult to avoid all animal products as a practical matter. Gary Francione addresses this same point in his excellent book, *Introduction to Animal Rights*:

...assume that we find that the local water company employs child labor and we object to child labor. Are we obligated to die of dehydration because the water company has chosen to violate the rights of children? No, of course not. We would be obligated to support the abolition of this use of children, but we would not be obligated to die. Similarly, we should join together collectively and demand an end to animal exploitation, but we are not obligated to accept animal exploitation or forego any benefits that it might provide.[19]

The important point here is to recognize when you're in a situation in which consuming the product that contains animal ingredients is unavoidable versus when it is avoidable. We can't stress enough that most people can easily avoid animal products and foods containing them — even when they're on vacation in Paris. Yet, we don't want anyone thinking that to be a "good" vegan, they need to forego medicine that has been prescribed to them by a doctor,[20] or that they need to give up their daily commute because of the by-product in the tires of the bus they're riding in.

IT ISN'T VEGETARIANISM

Earlier in this chapter, we explained why vegetarianism is a poor response to the problem of animal exploitation. If you're still not convinced, you need to stop deluding yourself: there is no way to logically or morally reconcile vegetarianism that includes animal products with an animal rights position. If you're currently a vegetarian, you probably think we're just moralizing assholes who want to judge you, but we assure you, that's not the case. We don't want to judge you at all — we just want you to go vegan, and to stop trying to justify your animal abuse as somehow good for animals. Any way that you can think to justify vegetarianism as "good for the animals" is a way that must, by its nature, be completely flawed. To do such a thing, you either would have to ignore the notion that animals have the right to be free from exploitation, or your idea of a what a right is so severely impoverished as to mean almost nothing. Or, we suppose, you could simply favor a different set of fundamental rights for yourself and creatures like you, while supporting a different set of rights for animals. But to do this would be flawed, too, because in the respects that animals are like us — insofar as they can breathe, have mental processes, feel pain, and have emotions — they deserve the same basic and essential protections we do. We're not saying that animals should have every single one of the same rights humans do — for example, it'd not be useful for cows to vote, or to have free speech — but we are saying that animals deserve the same fundamental rights that we humans enjoy, most notably, the right not to be the property of another, and the right not to be used exclusively as the means for another's ends. Since we're similar in those essential respects, any lines drawn that allow us to violate those essential rights of animals are wholly arbitrary. Though we go into this in a lot more depth in Chapter 2, this idea of rights is important to note, because it may help you to think through the following hypothetical, designed to drive home this point.

Gourmet, foodie-type assholes — many of whom have since given up life's real adventures and now consume their way through "exotic" foods in search of the next thrill — are always on the lookout for more obscure foods to consume, probably so they can brag to their friends about how incomprehensibly amazing and daring their palates are. For the sake of this hypothetical, let's assume that in some alternate universe, Anthony Bourdain finds the freshest-tasting and most intensely amazing milk he has ever had while doing one of his ridiculous food tours. His army of foodie toadies, many of whom are reduced to living vicariously through the adventures of their badass hero, see him sample it on TV, and immediately want to buy gallons of it to impress their friends at their upcoming dinner parties, cost be damned. AsswholePaycheck, an alternate-universe natural and organic foods conglomerate that sells only the highest quality foods, immediately takes up the cause, and promises to stock it at each of their stores within a few weeks. The milk, however, is produced by human females who have been genetically selected over many generations for their ability to produce the greatest amounts of milk. Through the many generations of selective breeding for the sole trait of milk production, these women have largely become severely mentally disabled. Though they still feel all human emotions and they possess rudimentary speech, they have essentially been turned into machines for the production of milk. In this horrible alternate universe, human slavery is legal, and so these women are owned outright by investors who offer them a comfortable place to sleep, plenty of food, and minimal entertainment consisting of re-runs of *Everybody Loves Raymond* and the ability to listen to any album at any time from the entire Dave Matthews Band back catalog. (We had to throw in the stuff about Raymond and Dave in case the hypothetical wasn't scary enough.) Though the women live what appears to be a comfortable life, once the women turn 35, the investors know that their productivity declines very rapidly, so the women are humanely and painlessly killed in a way which is, to them, very much like taking a pleasant nap.

Now, we're pretty sure that none of the above would stop most foodies — and especially not Anthony Bourdain — from drinking the milk, but did anything in the hypothetical make you uncomfortable? Like most people who possess even the most basic moral machinery, you probably (hopefully?!) found it highly objectionable that mentally-disabled women were used to produce milk, that they were owned outright as slaves, and that they only had *Everybody Loves Raymond* and Dave Matthews Band albums for occupying themselves. If you were bothered by the basic dynamic of the hypothetical, it is probably because you are not a sociopath and have a fervent moral belief that humans should not be exploited or owned as slaves. We agree. But if you found yourself feeling uneasy or angry about the alternate universe, the question you must ask yourself is this: why is it okay to do it to cows, but not to humans? In the above case, these humans were brought into existence and bred solely for this purpose, much like cows are. In the above example, these humans were not of "normal" human intelligence, and neither are cows. In the above example, the humans could feel emotions and pain, much like cows can. So, in all the ways that it really matters, the humans and the cows are pretty much alike in the hypothetical. For most of you who aren't suffering from some kind of antisocial personality disorder, there's a deep moral sense that treating human beings this way is wrong. If you can feel this moral sense for humans, why not also feel it for cows?

IT ISN'T HATING FOOD

For people who allegedly hate food, vegans sure do blog about it a lot. Go on out to the wilds of the Intertubes and have a look: there are approximately 8,234,587[21] vegan food blogs where authors describe the recipes they've prepared and the foods they've tried, usually with pictures. Apart from learning that some vegans are fantastic cooks — and noticing that others who think they are probably are not, at least judging by the piles of grayish mush they decide to post pictures of on their blogs — we've discovered that many vegans eat an incredibly wide variety of foods that draw on multiple cooking traditions. Vegans with culinary talent have re-imagined all kinds of dishes from the meat-and-potatoes-centric cuisines of Europe and the Americas, as well as looking to the many vegan-friendly cooking traditions of Asia and the Middle East for inspiration. While not all vegans eat such a wide variety of foods, we and many vegans we know love to eat from a wide swath of global cuisines, and for most of us, we really only began to explore these options in earnest after going vegan. Contrary to the notions that some people have, we vegans actually love to eat, we just prefer to eat things that didn't used to be a someone.

IT ISN'T ABOUT OPRAH

If you happened to be hanging around with anyone involved in the animal rights movement in May 2008, you could be forgiven for wondering if people who cared about animals had morphed into some millenarian UFO cult whose space-faring brethren were finally ready to liberate humanity from its ghastly chains.[22] The jubilation, exuberant glee, and fervent belief that things would change now — finally! — seemed to spread faster than a bad case of Norovirus on a cruise ship, especially within the more irrational quarters of the movement. No, animal rights activists had not been given a billion dollars by some über-wealthy foundation to promote veganism intelligently. No, we had not received a message from the spaceship behind the comet that would suddenly make everyone renounce their omnivorism. No, friends, something much more magical and fantastic happened: Oprah Winfrey went vegan! Rejoice, rejoice, rejoice!

Or not.

While we thought it was generally a good thing that someone so prominent decided to go vegan, Oprah was not the best role model for sensible veganism. It was pretty obvious that Oprah's movement to veganism was a temporary "diet," rather than the real and lasting changes that we think are most important. From the start, Oprah talked about going on her vegan "cleanse," as if every vegan was a vegan just to keep themselves shitting on schedule. Don't get us wrong: shitting frequently is good for your health, and we're never ones to deny the obvious gastrointestinal benefits of veganism, but we're ethical vegans, and so, for us, the only reason to go vegan and stay vegan is the moral imperative to stop treating animals as instruments for our ends. While Oprah did make some insinuations that her spiritual guru Eckhardt Tolle got her to think about going vegan for the sake of animals, by all accounts, she dropped her vegan try-out pretty promptly, probably leaving viewers everywhere a bit confused about what veganism really is. Taking Oprah as a role model, you could be forgiven for thinking that veganism is something you did to clean out your colon rather than something that you do to respect the inherent personhood of animals.

Clearly, Oprah was not the fabled savior that so many imagined her to be. If she got anyone to go vegan, they probably quit when she did, and apart from getting the word "vegan" in a bit wider circulation, we're not convinced Oprah did much of anything more with her "cleanse," with the exception of clogging up a few more golden toilets around her mansion. In fact, Oprah was probably even kind of negative for veganism on the whole, because she made people think that veganism is even more difficult than it really is. It is easy to imagine the vast numbers of people out there who said to themselves, "Wow, Oprah has a team of chefs and coaches and spiritual gurus helping her, and she can't even stick with it, so it must be impossible."

In this Oprah saga, we see not only the dangers of having idols — a subject about which we will spill significant ink in the coming pages — but also the dangers of going vegan for the wrong reasons. Though we honestly wish that everyone were vegan, there are some people who end up vegan and are not really ready to be. As a result, they often become the dreaded "ex-vegan," a special breed of annoyance for whom Dante should have invented the tenth circle of Hell. The by-product of poor reasons for going vegan, the "ex-vegan" is often the person who is lurking behind every corner, ready to undermine you by loudly proclaiming in some whiny cry just how "hard" veganism is, and how they "tried to be vegan" but couldn't keep with it for whatever reason. It could be that they missed ham or cheese or bacon. It could be that they felt that they lacked vigor without the blood of dead animals dripping down their chins. It could be that they simply couldn't stand the occasional minor inconveniences. Whatever the reason, these people not only make you look like the freak in the room, they also unhelpfully reaffirm every belief that every non-vegan has about veganism: that it is too hard, too radical, too weird, and not worth the trouble.

Going vegan isn't that hard in the scheme of things, but it is a big step that, if taken seriously, requires you to make changes in your daily life. Some of these changes seem relatively big and some are small and simple, but if your heart isn't in it — if you aren't vegan for the right reasons — the changes are ultimately going to fall by the wayside. As we see it, there are a bunch of wrong reasons to become vegan, but all of them revolve around one's heart, ethics, and principles not being at the core of this all-important choice.

FAME AND FRIENDS

People in the animal rights movement got all excited over Oprah's foray into veganism because they figured that her fan base would go vegan along with her. And probably, some of them did, for a time at least. For a few weeks in 2008, our vegan ranks likely swelled with die-hard Oprahites, many of whom, reverently clutching glossy copies of the latest *O Magazine*, devoted themselves to a vegan "cleanse" along with the celebrity they worshipped. Most of these people probably are not vegan now, likely having suffered through a few colon-blowing days or weeks of eating what they imagined "healthy" and "cleansing" vegan foods to be. For her part, Oprah valiantly took one for the team by having her food prepared for her by professional chefs, consulting with her sundry spiritual gurus, and, on at least one show, thanking hummus personally for "coming to the table."

We aren't trying to diss on the deliciousness of hummus. We're always grateful when hummus comes to our table, but we're not so sure about these disillusioned people who went vegan because Oprah did. Could their hearts have really been in it, or were they doing it because their celebrity hero did? And though we're picking on Oprah for the moment, it is just as easy to look at other vegan celebrities whose followers go vegan for the wrong reasons. There are plenty of brainless straight-edgers who go vegan only because Earth Crisis said they should, just as there are surely some Coldplay fans who, like, have to totally go vegan because, um, Chris Martin like totally is, OMG!!! Regardless, going vegan in an attempt to be like your favorite celebrity is just setting yourself up for a world of hurt.

Similarly, celebrity or not, going vegan to emulate someone who you think is cool is ridiculously stupid. It is also not advisable to go vegan in order to impress a lover, or to try to get laid. Unbelievable as it may be for you horny, single vegans out there suffering away in your lonely, masturbatory Hells in rural Wyoming or wherever you are, some people actually do go vegan as a ploy to get into the pants of a certain special someone, or to curry favor towards such ends. We're not religious fundamentalists, and we don't really care what you and any other number of consenting adults decide to do with your respective junks behind closed doors. We also know that you need to get your freak on and all that, and we'd never want to deny you the many pleasures that human sexuality can offer — though we do ask both figuratively and literally that you don't fuck with the animals.[23] All we really want is for veganism to be something that means something, and for that to happen, people have to take it seriously, and not use it to manipulate others for social or sexual ends. If you're going vegan to make friends, to impress someone, or to get some action, U R DOIN IT WRONG. Don't bother trying to be something that you're not. It is probably quite painful to live a life that you aren't really into, and you can only pretend to be something that you aren't for so long before the veneer wears off. Plus, relationships of all stripes do best when honesty is the currency of the realm, and you'll be happier if you realize that the best friends and the best lovers are people who just accept you for who you are. It might be best to think of it like this: if veganism actually and honestly is a part of who you are, and it feels right to you even if all of your friends are doing it, then embrace it. If you want to go vegan because someone you respect is vegan, and you understand what veganism is about and it makes sense to you, embrace it. But don't use it as a tool for manipulating anyone, including yourself. You only hurt yourself, you hurt your friends and/or lovers, and you hurt the cause of veganism.

Whatever the case — whether you're trying to be like a super-star, or to make yourself more acceptable to friends and lovers — in the previous instances, the motivation for going vegan is too externalized and too weak; you cannot go vegan to please another, or to try to become something or someone that you're not. You can only go vegan and stay vegan if you truly believe in the choice yourself. Doing it any other way is just a quick road to frustration, upset, and a miserable life of ex-vegandom.

IT ISN'T SOMETHING YOU DO TO ASSERT JUST HOW UNIQUE AND INDIVIDUAL A SNOWFLAKE YOU ARE

It's like totally hard to do anything that's original anymore. You get a fixed gear bike that you don't know how to ride properly, and next thing you know, everyone on your block has one, and you're all colliding into one another and blowing stop signs because your neighbors don't really know how to make them stop, either. You start wearing trucker hats, and then discover that the trend died sometime in the very early-oughts. You hunt down Animal Collective's *Merriweather Post Pavilion* on 180-gram vinyl, and then find out, much to your surprise, that your roommate has already colonized that particular corner of unique. Though it sucks, the truth is, if you can imagine anything that you think is unique, the odds are good that someone has probably already done it. Worse yet, there's probably some Prada-clad overpaid consultant sitting in a corporate marketing department somewhere in New York at this very moment who is hiring models to do a shoot so that his mega-ultra-corp employer can figure out a way to sell you more stupid shit you probably don't need.

The hunt for the ever-elusive piece of kit to make you über-rad is harder now than it has ever been. And who knows what's coming next? If you asked us, we'd never have guessed that people would be dumb enough to dress like lumberjacks while strolling about the Lower East Side in New York, or that people who know nothing about bikes would suddenly start riding ones that last saw their best days on a velodrome in the '84 Olympics. We don't know what's coming next, and really, we don't care. But we do want to dissuade you from using veganism as part of your little ensemble of radical uniqueness. Being vegan doesn't make you ironic, genuine, or radical. Yeah, we know... veganism can make you a fabulous pain in the ass sometimes. It can make you look "alternative" or "green" or even "sensitive." Hell, it probably compliments your lifestyle better than that new courier bag you just got that cups your ass ever-so-gracefully when you're jetting off on your bike to your next $50 haircut appointment. But here's the thing: going vegan isn't really about your identity. It is about taking a stand against exploitation, and demanding that animals be regarded as something more than mere means to our ends. If you are a vegan, and it happens to compliment the rest of your lifestyle, bully for you — consider it a bonus. If you're just using veganism to look "alt," then fuck off elsewhere and find a new trend to hop on, poseur.

IT ISN'T BEING AFRAID OF THE WORD "VEGAN"

Some people have the idea that the word "vegan" is scary, non-inclusive, elitist, and alienating, and to combat this, some vegans actually avoid calling themselves vegans, referring to themselves instead as "veggies," or saying that they eat a "plant-based diet." With so many people so con-fused about what veganism is, we understand why people might do such a thing, and we even get why new vegans in particular may be tempted to downplay their own veganism, lest they appear to be too weird. Unfortunately, none of these strategies are all that useful, and instead of combating the problem of people not understanding veganism, they quietly reinforce the misunderstanding by relegating veganism to obscurity. Unless we take the time to educate others about veganism and why we are vegan, the elegant and powerful message of veganism will remain misunderstood, and our goal of abolishing animal exploitation will be deferred.

To take up one of the main points of veganism — to serve as a kind of public reminder that all is not well with how we relate to animals as humans — people have to know that we're vegan, not that we're eating a "plant-based diet," or Flying Spaghetti Monster forbid, that we are "veggies." In reference to a human being, what the fuck is a "veggie," anyway? Is it a cute vegetarian? A vegan? An ovo-lacto vegetarian? Either a vegan or a vegetarian? And who would be proud to refer to themselves using terminology that young children use to talk about the green stuff on their dinner plates? Add to this the idea that if you call yourself a "veggie," you are sending the message that you have little higher brain function, and the problems of calling yourself a "veggie" become immediately apparent.

Though not as cloying as the term "veggie," "plant-based diet" suffers from similar problems if you're opting for it over "vegan." First, "plant-based diet" sounds like a term you'd use if you were David Attenborough narrating a BBC nature special on the habits of a rare vegetable-eating animal. The term is descriptive, but cold and scientific, and it is a mouth-ful that does not lend itself to everyday use. To take just one example, is someone who eats a plant-based diet a plant-based dieter, or does that same person have to say that she "eats a plant-based diet?" Either way, those descriptions lack the simplicity and ease of "vegan." Second, those vegans who describe themselves as eating a "plant-based diet" — the plant-based-dieter vegans, if you will — reinforce the idea that vegetarianism is merely a "diet" to go on to lower your cholesterol, or to squeeze into that pair of jeans that make your ass look hot. Veganism actually can have wonderful benefits, which may include a lower blood cholesterol count and an overall improvement in the attractiveness of your ass, but these are selling points that are largely tangential to the main issue of ethical veganism, which is taking a stand against the systemic exploitation of animals in our world. Veganism isn't a "diet." It is a way of living that focuses on according animals their due right as fellow sentient beings.

When it comes down to it, people need to know that you're a vegan. If people don't know what veganism is, and they seem genuinely curious, tell them. If you're afraid that the very idea of calling yourself a "vegan" might make others wary of you, or scare people off, the solution isn't to run from veganism. The solution is to live your life in a way that proves to people that veganism is not the equivalent of joining a cult.

Impoverished Veganism and the Need for Social Change

A few years ago, before we were even vegan, we gave up eating Oreos.

In case you have a different corporate hegemon where you live and have no clue what an Oreo is, just imagine two chocolaty discs compressed around a dense, fatty blob of white sugar, and you're pretty much there. The whole cookie together is 53 calories of sugar, fat, and chemical food additives, and people rarely eat just one. Overly sweet yet completely delicious, the Oreo, like so much junk food, registers positive hits on the primitive parts of our brain that were used to encourage us to eat lots of this stuff, largely to guard against conditions of uneven food supply that were a normal part of human evolutionary history. As a result, there's a part of all of us that loves sweet, fatty stuff like this, a neurochemical hold-out from our hunter-gatherer days, before we could count on taking a run down to the grocery store when we needed anything. A little piece of corporate-derived cookie-like crack, the Oreo seems designed to take calories from the package and load them directly on your ass, gut, or wherever it is that you happen to put on weight when you consume too much.

While rumor has it that at least in the USA the ubiquitous sandwich cookie is made with vegan ingredients, Oreos are just too delicious a vehicle for the delivery of the very things we needed not eat much of, like fat, sugar, and who the hell knows what kinds of chemical preservatives. Thus, largely in deference to our health, we cut off the Oreo jones suddenly one day, never to return to the land of the corporate crack-cookie.

We've been Oreo-clean for many years now, but on occasion, the siren call of corporate-produced junk food is indeed strong in our ears, and on the rarest and most unique of occasions when the stars are aligned just so, we wander to that no-man's land in the middle of the grocery store, to those inner aisles where nothing is fresh, nothing is healthy, and nothing is really worth eating. There, nestled comfortably among Nutter Butters, ChipsAhoy! and other American industrial cookie output, one can now find a dizzying array of Oreos, greatly expanded from the former simplicity of regular and double-stuff. Now, there's some kind of blonde-hued Oreo — clearly a sign that the End Times are near — an Incredible Hulk Oreo, vibrant with green filling, and even a despair-flavored Oreo commemorating Robert Falcon Scott's failed North Pole expedition of 1910-13 (okay, not really. But seriously, the variety is almost this absurdly large.)

By now you're probably thinking to yourself "Fuck this Oreo shit(e) already, I bought the book to read about veganism. Get on with it!" Well, fear not, there is a point. Since giving up Oreos all those years ago, we can honestly report that there has been no discernible decline in Oreo supply at local grocery stores. If anything, the variety of Oreos has grown by leaps and bounds in some kind of genius marketing coup that is comprehensible only to the evil cookie cartels that devise these things. There's obviously no reason why this glut of cookies should be surprising: after all, only two of us gave up Oreos, and production of Oreos has continued unabated since the day we quit. Owned by Altria, a company whose name sounds more like a disease than a business entity — "Oh my God! You have ALTRIA?! How much longer do you have to live?" — the Oreo brand is a multinational power-house that sells tons of cookies a year to millions of people around the world. There's simply no sensible reason to believe that the lone action of the two of us would make a whit of difference in the production of these cookies. But what would happen if instead of just us two giving up Oreos, ten million of us gave up Oreos? Further still, what would happen if the ten million of us who gave up Oreos organized with other Oreo-boycotters, and educated people about what perceived the problems to be with Oreos? Let's also assume that through that education and outreach, each of us con-vinced a dozen other people to give them up, and that dozen also began educating others. Pretty soon, Altria's cookie portfolio would be limping along minus one of its star players, and we'd actually have a group of people organized around the common goal of Oreo-boycotting. To do this would prob-ably not be all that hard, provided we were thoughtful about how we did it, and provided we had a convincing argument or story to sell our activism.

By now, it should be clear that the moral of this story isn't really about Oreos. Instead, our point is that veganism can only find its fullest and most effective expression as an objec-tion to the exploitation of animals when all of us who are vegan do the hard work of educating, building connections with others, and moving out beyond the limited confines of our own lives. Individuals being vegan in their own lives are the building-blocks of this movement, and we very much believe that the veganism of any single individual is vital, yet we need to move beyond what we call "impoverished veg-anism," or the notion that veganism is solely about what we do or do not consume. At this point in history, and probably for the rest of our lives at the very least, individual change is a necessary but not sufficient condition for a successful vegan movement that abolishes of animal slavery. To put it another way, going vegan is the absolute minimum you can do, but because of the David and Goliath proportions of the battle, we cannot afford the luxury of mere consumerism. If we are ever going to defeat the multibillion- dollar global behemoths that exploit animals for profit, we must also be activists and educators, writers and thinkers, and organizers and protesters. We have to know our arguments well, and talk to people about them convincingly and logically. We have to do the incredibly important but sometimes boring and inglorious work that goes along with growing the roots of a real social movement. And most importantly for a world where everything is instant and we all hate to wait for any-thing, we have to learn to take a long-term view, and concep-tualize this as a struggle that may not be won in our lifetimes. Social change can move at what seems like a glacial pace, but shifts in societal consciousness do obviously happen. As ethical vegans, it is our job to do what we can to bring this shift about in the social and cultural understandings of animal-human relations. Only then can these understandings be translated into material changes that will end the com-modification of animals.

Creating a movement that has broad social power and an even broader social presence requires moving beyond mere consumerism. Admittedly, this will be a challenge. We have to change the world around us while also changing ourselves, or to put it another way, we have to live the revolution, and that's never easy. At this point, one of the biggest hurdles in living the revolution is that consumerism is quite comfortable and familiar for those of us who have money and live in capi-talist countries. The purported solution to problems ranging from defeating greenhouse gas emissions to ending slavery in the chocolate trade, "voting" with one's money has become a commonplace stand-in for effective and lasting social protest. In this model, citizens gain the full right to articulate how they want the world to be only if they can spend their way towards that end. As very real and very potent desires for social change are channeled into buying one set of stuff instead of another set of stuff, the social energy and vibrancy of a movement gets drained, shunted off into a market activity that can be easily managed and steered by those in power. Instead of being an activist, you become a customer. Instead of being a citizen, you are a consumer. Instead of getting a vote that really matters, you get to spend your money as you please. Oh, and of course, all of this presumes that you actually have money to spend — we wouldn't want to give too much of this power to poor people now, would we?

Obviously, we believe that the stuff you buy is important, or we wouldn't go to the lengths that we go to in this book to help you avoid products laced with cruelty. Plus, to deny that consumption matters would just be dumb. Our point, instead, is that we have to be more than what we buy or do not buy. In the impoverished veganism that relies on consumerism as the lone vehicle for social action, we all end up sitting alone in each of our homes, eating our cool-ass vegan cupcakes, surfing the web for new vegan message shirts to really stick it to The Man, and ordering the newest pleather boots so we can look rad as fuck. As a result, we've constructed an identity for ourselves that we're mostly performing through the stuff we buy. While the society we live in encourages us to pursue our identities through our material possessions, no other social movement that we are aware of has effectively made any real, lasting changes exclusively by having people in the movement buy or not buy particular things as the primary mode of social activism. Though overused to the point of cliché in Lefty circles, the example of Martin Luther King easily springs to mind.

During his famous 1963 speech at the Lincoln Memorial in Washington, D.C., King did not encourage people to go out and buy a more equitable America. Instead, he told them that they could not walk alone, that they had to work together to achieve the dream of freedom.

We cannot walk alone anymore. If we're going to make any change at all, we need to move beyond the stuff, and take a public role in helping to push our respective societies towards an understanding of how animals deserve person-hood. We can only do this through a concentrated collective action that leverages the talents that each and every one of us has — a point which we'll return to later. If we fail to build a genuine abolitionist social movement with veganism at its core, we will be damned to near-total irrelevance, which is a horrendous, crying shame, because everyday vegans like you are the most powerful outreach tool in this long and entrenched struggle for the abolition of animal slavery.

Embrace Your Vegan Freakdom

The first step towards building a genuine social movement of ethical vegans is embracing your inner vegan freakdom. Somehow, in this incredibly strange world where it is absolutely normal to gnaw on the dismembered body parts of other sentient beings, you've managed to overcome the overwhelming cultural and social messages that say that animals are ours to do with as we please. This is a powerful realization, and now that you have come to this realization, your conscience will not likely rest. Being vegan is the first and most important step towards achieving justice for ani-mals, and of living your life in a way that fits with your beliefs. Yes, at times, you might be made to feel stupid, radical, or even insane. People almost certainly will make fun of you or marginalize you, and you should expect at least some kind of backlash as you take a stand against the accepted social order. This is all a small price to pay, however, for living fully and honestly with yourself and with animals, and for being part of a movement that will someday achieve liberation for beings whose exploitation and enslavement is severe and entrenched. If we all work hard enough and give of ourselves to educate others through nonviolent activism, there will come a day when human society will recognize its wrongs with regard to animals. When we look back, which side are you going to be on? Are you going to be one of the ethical vegans, or are you going to be one of those who held up progress towards a more just world?

Be on the right side of history: be vegan.

Notes to Chapter 1

1   Seriously! 21 percent of people in a poll done by the Roper organization believe that people are being abducted by aliens. See this URL for details: http://www.scifi.com/ufo/roper/05.html.

2   Julia Preston, "After Iowa Raid, Immigrants Fuel Labor Inquiries," *New York Times*, July 27, 2008.

3   Donald Watson, *The Vegan News* (Quarterly Magazine of the Non-Dairy Vegetarians), http://www.ukveggie.com/vegan_news/.

4   Different breeds are bred for different purposes, often dictated by the desired efficiencies of the producers. For example, so-called "broiler" chickens grow rapidly and gain weight fast so that they can be brought to market faster, turning a quicker profit for the producer. Egg-layers are bred for egg production, and so are not suitable for meat production. This kind of distinction is also present in cattle, where some breeds are exclusively bred for milking, while others are bred exclusively for the quality of their meat.

5   It also bears mentioning (since many people forget this fact) that cows just don't automatically give milk. Like humans, cows must be impregnated and give birth before they will produce milk, so dairy cows are in a constant cycle of being pregnant, giving birth, and producing milk before they become unproductive and are sent to slaughter. The calves, a "by-product" of dairy production, either become future dairy cows or veal.

6   Ursula LeGuin, *The Dispossessed* (New York: EOS, 1974).

7   For those of you who aren't down with the lingo, according to the authoritative source on all things slangy, Urbandictionary.com, an "Alt-Bro is much like the Dave Matthews listening, sandal wearing Bro of the 90's, only wears tight pants, and only alternative music." http://www.urbandictionary.com/define.php?term=Alt-Bro

8   http://clinicaltrials.gov/ct2/show/NCT00360919?cond=%22Food+Habits%22&rank=1

9   All figures from http://www.nutritiondata.com.

10 It can also help you save money. If you go to the grocery store with a list of what you need and a plan for a few days worth of meals, the odds are that you will be less tempted to buy things that you don't really need and may not end up using.

11   We didn't call the press we founded Tofu Hound for nothing. Every time we open a package of tofu in our household, our two dogs come running, demanding to be paid their royalties for the naming rights.

12   There is one thing, though, about our forums: because of the large number of spammers and scammers, we require users to write an introduction detailing their path to veganism, and we ask that anyone seeking membership already be vegan or significantly on the way to veganism. Other forums have less strict entry requirements, so look around if this bothers you, or if you're not vegan yet.

13   Say hi to us on Twitter, or follow us if you want. Our Twitter URLs are http://twitter.com/veganfreak and http://twitter.com/pleather.

14   A good place to start with research on this is *The China Study: The Most Comprehensive Study of Nutrition Ever Conducted and the Startling Implications for Diet, Weight Loss, and Long-Term Health*, by T. Colin Campbell and Thomas M. Campbell. 1st ed. (Dallas, TX: BenBella Books, 2005). Neal Barnard has also authored several books that provide extensive details on the connections between veganism and long-term health.

15   Neal Barnard, *Dr. Neal Barnard's Program for Reversing Diabetes: The Scientifically Proven System for Reversing Diabetes without Drugs.* (New York: Rodale, 2008).

16   More on this in Chapter 2.

17   More on this later too.

18   But in all truth, Peter Singer and his act-utilitarian counterparts do not care about rights for animals in the least — a point we will return to in greater depth in Chapter 2.

19   Gary L. Francione, *Introduction to Animal Rights: Your Child or the Dog?* (Philadelphia: Temple University Press, 2000), 118.

20   This sounds crazy, but you'd be surprised how many emails we get from people asking us if they should take their prescribed medicines because they were tested on animals. Our answer is always this: take it if your doctor says so. If you aren't sure about the utility of any particular medicine, get a second opinion from a different doctor.

21   In case you've lost your hyperbole meter, this number is completely fabricated to make a point, though as of mid-2009, Google does return something like 18,800,000 hits for the search term "vegan food blog," so perhaps it isn't the incredible hyperbole we imagine it to be!

22   Come to think of it, you could be forgiven if wondering if the animal rights movement is a cult, especially when you see some of the ridiculous shit PETA does on a daily basis.

23   Peter Singer, in an article in the online magazine *Nerve*, talked about the common cultural taboo over human-animal sexuality. In discussing this, Singer describes how we've all been audience to a dog "vigorously rubbing its penis against" visitors, but that "in private not everyone objects to being used by her or his dog in this way, and occasionally mutually satisfying activities may develop." To be blunt, we think this is fucked up. Though the dog seeks out the behavior, there is no reason to presume that it is acceptable as a moral matter to allow the dog to become an instrument of human sexual pleasure, regardless of what the dog gets out of it; such behavior objectifies the dog in a world where animals already are objects to just about everyone. To take an analogous example, if a child who did not know better rubbed their genitals on an adult caretaker and the caretaker allowed a "mutually satisfying" activity to develop, we'd question whether that caretaker should be allowed around children. To be clear, we're not implying that Singer is a pedophile, but we certainly wouldn't let him around our fur family. Check out Singer's article yourself at http://www.nerve.com/Opinions/Singer/heavyPetting/.

CHAPTER 2

BOB AND JENNA SOLVE
THE NORTH KOREA PROBLEM

WHEN WE SAT DOWN AND STARTED PLANNING the second edition of this book, we had some relatively modest goals for what the book might accomplish. First, we figured that the deft wit, acerbic and biting prose, and Vulcan-like logic of our book would drive a small but significant part of the global masses to embrace veganism, leading to a giant Tsunami-like vegan wave that would sweep all into its massive sway. Second, we imagined that once the Tsunami crashed down about humanity, we'd pull apart an ethically bankrupt set of industries that profit from the suffering of animals. And third, because we figured that the first two points were, like, so *totally* doable (dude — we do shit like this *before you even wake up* most days), and because Bob has ADHD, hates being bored, and is not so great at setting realistic goals, we decided we'd also set out to solve the North Korea problem.

Yeahhhhh.

Okay, admittedly, this is all tinged with just the tiniest bit of hyperbole. We do want everyone to go vegan. We do want to pull apart the ethically bankrupt animal exploitation industries. And as for North Korea, who wouldn't want to help

Dear Leader get along with the rest of the world? But knowing what we know about our limitations, we'll be happy if a few of you go vegan. (We'd also be happy if we could do something about the North Korea problem, but that'll probably have to wait until our next book.)

So, if we can't do anything about North Korea, you may be wondering why we'd ever do something cheap like titling our chapter with such a nice, neat declarative sentence that could never, ever possibly be true. Our reasons are simple. Going to press, we were stuck on what to call this chapter. We had many ideas, kicked around over many months, but all were ultimately unsatisfactory. (This writing books stuff sounds like so much fun until you actually have to sit down and do it. SIGH.) Then, at the very last minute, with our publisher breathing hot breath down our sweaty necks, we needed to come up with something. We could have done the totally obvious thing and used a descriptive title, but we wanted something that was a bit of a non sequitur to get you thinking.

Being huge fans of the TV show *It's Always Sunny in Philadelphia,* (and yes, OMFG, Bob and Jenna own a TV and we watch it and we're such tools of consumerist society!) we decided to shamelessly adapt the title of one of their episodes for our chapter. We also were thinking of calling the chapter "Bob and Jenna Go All Animal Rights All Over Everybody's Ass," which has clear advantages, but also some clear disadvantages the implications of which are best left to the ever-dirty imaginations of our more gutter-minded readers.

To sum up: this chapter has nothing to do with North Korea or Kim Jong Il. Nor does it have anything to do with us doing anything all over anyone's ass. Instead, this chapter gives you a basic overview to understand why animal rights matter, why extending them to animals would be consistent as a moral matter, and why consistency matters in our actions and outreach. Please recognize that this chapter is intended to provide only the most broad of outlines of what are fairly well developed theoretical frameworks. We hate to assign home-work, but it is our sincere belief that vegans should be well educated about animal rights issues. We give you the basics here, but there's really no substitute for doing more reading yourself, and learning to grasp some of these ideas on your own. If you want somewhere to begin once you're done this chapter, we think you should start with Gary L. Francione's book *Introduction to Animal Rights: Your Child or the Dog*. Bob's book *Making A Killing: The Political Economy of Animal Rights* is a good companion to Francione's book, since it explains and extends certain key aspects of Francione's thinking. Whatever you read, we think you should read about these ideas and get as familiar with them as you can. Contrary to the rampant anti-intellectual gripes that you'll see out there in the animal rights movement about how theory is a luxury when so many animals are dying, the ideas matter a great deal. Ideas matter because ideas guide action, and without underlying ideas and principles, you run the risk of doing things that may now or in the future work against the very things you are trying to achieve. Thus, you should learn the theory before you get into action — by doing so, you can make your efforts all that more powerful. Though some people would say that we don't have the luxury of theory, we'd say that we don't have the luxury of ignoring it. It is essential to our veganism.

With all that said, we now turn to a discussion of the rights of our chlorophyll-laden friends, the plants.

SURELY, FEW ARE THE VEGANS who have been vegan any significant amount of time who have not yet heard someone confidently announce that eating plants was some kind of grave social and moral injustice, because plants have feelings. Most of the low-grade morons who manage to come up with this kind of dim-witted response to veganism also tend to be a bit too dumb to know that not only are they not as brilliant as they think they are for coming up with it, but also that they're hardly the first person to have thought of it. Resisting the temptation to say "thank you for raising that point, genius! Let me ring up the Nobel folks and make sure that you get that award you've deserved all this time," is always hard. Sometimes, it isn't even worth holding back, because it is clear that your interlocutor himself has the IQ of the cabbage in your coleslaw. When confronted with such aggressive stupidity, you really should ask yourself if the battle is worth your time or effort.

On some occasions, though, the question about why we vegans care so much about the rights of animals and not so much about the rights of plants is one that deserves your honest and careful consideration, because the answer is ultimately telling about the ethics behind the decision to go vegan. (And no, it isn't that we vegans hate plants, though there may be a few extra-surly types in our ranks who hate plants just because they hate *everything*.) Though we like to poke fun at the snarky saviors for all of plant-kind, there are some who genuinely want to understand why we have an ethical issue with eating animals and a completely clear conscience about eating plants. While some people are just fools who want to waste your time and have a laugh at your expense, others aren't, and it isn't usually hard to tell the difference by the sincerity of the question.

It may be hard to believe that anyone could ask such a question seriously, but some people do, and when they do, you need to remember that they're merely reflecting the view of the dominant culture in which we all live. To the ethical vegan, a steak is a bloody piece of flesh, extracted from a suffering being who should have every right to be free of that suffering. To the meat eater, however, a steak is a delicious delicacy, and to most meat eaters, the distant echo of the slaughterhouse is quite far off indeed. For the everyday non-vegan, a steak is food just like a carrot is food. If you care about how one kind of food feels, why not care about how the other kind of food feels too?

Obviously, this is some wickedly bad logic, but such is what you'll have to face out there in the world. What people tend to forget when they buy their steaks, all nice and neat and wrapped up in cellophane and Styrofoam, is that animals are like us in a great many respects. Plants feel no pain, but animals surely do. Like you, animals have sensory organs, nervous systems, and pain receptors. Like you, many of the animals eaten by the rest of society are mammals. Like you, those very same animals want to be comfortable, free, and happy. Like you, many animals desire and seek out companionship. In their sentience, animals have subjective experiences that they remember, and there are many compelling reasons to assume that those experiences share at least some of the qualities that your own experiences do. As with you, they can have a good time of things, or a bad time of things. If you cause animals pain, they will react in much the same way you or I would react: they would try to get away from it, to distance themselves from whatever the cause was.

Looking at it from the plant side of things, if you try to cause broccoli some pain, you'll find out pretty quickly that if broccoli feels anything at all, it does a pretty crap job of showing it. Perhaps broccoli is just the quiet, stoic type who tries to keep a tough face through the pain, John Wayne style. Or, in the more likely scenario, broccoli doesn't actually feel a damn thing when you burn it. We do bump into a philosophical issue here called the "problem of other minds" which suggests that you can't ever have full and complete knowledge of what goes on in the head of another. When you stub your toe, we can't *really* know if you're feeling pain, even though you are hopping around on one foot screaming curse words that would make Charles Manson blush. Similarly, if we do something to broccoli that would cause a human or an animal pain — like burning it — we can't *really* know if broccoli is feeling pain or not. Still, you shouldn't make too much of the problem of other minds; in reality, it is really only a fun game for philosophy majors to kick around when they've smoked too much weed and want to feel deep. On a practical level, each of us goes through every single day of our lives not knowing with total certainty what is going on inside the heads of those around us, and most of us do just fine reading the external clues, particularly when it comes to something obvious like pain. Almost all of us can read the external cues well enough to see the problem, and maybe even to feel empathy for the person or animal experiencing the pain.

Broccoli provides us with none of these external indicators when it is harassed or subjected to various kinds of battery that would make a human being shudder. Broccoli has no sense organs, and seems to feel no pain. On top of this, broccoli doesn't evidence any desire for company with its little green broccoli comrades. Broccoli will never jump into your lap and purr (if it does, you probably need to re-up the meds). Broccoli provides no evidence that it has any subjective experiences. Broccoli is a living thing, but it isn't a living thing that seems to have a sense of itself, unlike the way that we do, and you do, and the animals that are eaten by people everyday do.

Broccoli, then, can't really be said to have anything that is remotely approaching sentience. It cannot feel pain; it seems to have no sense of itself; and, unless you want to resort to some rather esoteric philosophical or mystical doctrines, the idea that broccoli could have a subjective experience without nerves or sensory organs is laughable.

Such is the sad and frustrating state of the world that you have to be in the position of spelling this kind of obvious logic out to people, but it is important that you have a good grasp on this kind of logic, because you'll find these questions coming up over and over again. In this chapter, we give you some of the tools that you'll need to construct logical and compelling answers to similar questions that you'll no doubt be hearing in short order. The best way to do this is not to walk you step by step through every possible scenario, but rather, to give you the ability to think through your own answers yourself using the basic ideas that underlie the kinds of vegan choices we advocate. To do this, we provide you with an extremely basic primer on the abolitionist approach to animal rights and the kinds of activism that go along with this approach. As the name suggests, abolitionists wish to abolish animal exploitation — we don't want to regulate it or make it more humane. Having read and taught a great deal about these ideas, we are confident that the abolitionist theory of animal rights — pioneered by Professor Gary L. Francione — is the most compelling and logical way to understand and advocate for animal rights. Working from questions that hit at the heart of what it means to treat others morally, Francione gives us a perspective that is true to principles, a perspective that centers the powerful contribution that veganism and other forms of non-violent social activism can have in changing our world for the better.

Before we begin, though, we have one quick note. We understand that depending on where you are in your veganism, the notion of abolishing anything might sound radical to you. That's cool, and understandable, and we get it. When we went vegan, we approached many of these ideas with a bit of trepidation at first, and it took us time to come to see things differently. Overcoming a lifetime of understanding animals as something more than mere things takes time: while one part of your brain may grasp and agree with the logic, for some of you, there's another part that is made uncomfortable by the realizations that you're likely going to have. All we ask, then, is that you recognize this dynamic if you think it might be at play inside yourself. Give yourself time to think through these ideas, do some reading — what we give you here is only a cursory overview, and you really should consider reading more widely on the topic — and, most importantly, do the hard work of being honest with yourself about these ideas. It can take time to really see the necessity of veganism, but the sooner you see it and decide to make these positive changes in your life, the better — for you and for the animals. Along these lines, we hope that you will at least hear us out, and give us the chance to make the point before you close the book and storm off.[1]

Okay, enough of that — let's talk about a mean little shit named Simon.

Simon the Sadist

We already know that plants and animals are different, but what happens when we begin asking these same questions to compare animals and humans? In order to get to the heart of this question, in his book *Introduction to Animal Rights: Your Child or the Dog?* Gary Francione raises a compelling hypothetical that is worth considering. Let's say that there's a guy named Simon who — for his own pleasure and no other reason at all — enjoys burning his dog with a blowtorch. Yes, this is pretty screwed up, so it is reasonable to wonder: surely, Simon must be engaging in this kind of healthy, well-adjusted behavior for a reason, right? He might *say* that he's just doing it for fun, but no one is really that sick, right? Unfortunately, some people are that messed up, and Simon is to be counted among them. Simon is a sadist — he finds deep pleasure in inflicting pain on others, and dogs happen to be an easy target for him. Pressed at length, Simon's only real answer is that he's enjoying every minute of what he's doing. Put simply, Simon is what the experts would call a "sick fuck."

Now, let's say that Simon's case became national news. We've all seen news of horrible cases of animal abuse, ranging from the near-global furor over the Michael Vick pit bull abuse case to the occasional local news story in which local youth, working in their roles as budding serial killers, are found doing horrible things to kittens or puppies. For the sake of the hypothetical, let's say that Simon's neighbors complain about what he is doing, and Simon's case becomes a police matter. Much as happened in the Michael Vick case, Simon's case would likely garner the attention of a nation shocked by what we'd consider to be horribly unnecessary cruelty, and people from across the political spectrum and from just about every segment of society would rush out to denounce the barbarous acts. Apart from the truly sociopathic, no one would ever say that what Simon did was a good idea. Even his own defense attorney, having to stare down a news camera, would probably be stuck admitting just how screwed up Simon was.

Tuned into the ever-present idiot box, people would almost certainly catch up on the latest Simon the Sadist news over their evening dinners. Just before launching into an extended diatribe on how sick people are, one news viewer stabs a bit of a potato with his fork, and mushes it around in the bloody juices coming off of the steak he just ate. Another viewer, also ready to wonder aloud to his family at how someone can be so heartless, hungrily bites a chicken leg, sucking fervently on the joints and connective tissue for just a bit more flavor. Somewhere else out there in TV land, another viewer is lifting her third slice of extra-cheese pizza out of the box, catching the strings of hot mozzarella, and piling them on top of her slice so they don't go to waste; saddened by the news she sees as she's helping herself to her pizza, she has to put her food down and give her dog a little hug before she goes on. Like most other sane people who can empathize with other living beings, she can't imagine anyone ever being so completely heartless, and the idea that anyone would blow torch a dog, a creature like the one that she's hugging, a creature with whom she shares the joys and pleasures of life, brings her to tears. "Sick fucks," she thinks, as she's filled with a combination of rage and despair.

In its broadest outlines, the same essential scenario is repeated millions upon millions of times across the country as people tune into the TV news over their evening meal — an evening meal that is, almost universally, composed of some kind of animal flesh or animal excretion. Surely, over chicken legs, rump roasts, and baby-back ribs, Americans would express their outrage at such unnecessary cruelty. And in that expression, very few people would realize or even care that as they fill their stomachs with animal products, they are in no small part responsible for the visitation of acts of unimaginable cruelty on beings who are every bit as sentient as the dogs that Simon is burning for fun. Worse yet, their justifications for eating these animal products — just because they taste good, and are traditionally what people are used to eating — are essentially the same as Simon's when we get down to it.

In these two scenarios, we can begin to see what Francione calls our "moral schizophrenia" towards animals. While we can all agree that we should not impose unnecessary suffering on animals, we also, as a society, cause harm to animals for reasons that are a distant cry from "necessary." In Simon's case, we can all easily see that blow-torching a dog for mere pleasure is just plain unnecessary and cruel. No one, we reason, should be able to inflict that much suffering on an animal simply for their own pleasure — it seems gratuitous, unnecessary, a sick indulgence whose underlying condition is probably best dealt with by psychiatric professionals. Like the hypothetical diners above, we all tend to object to imposing that kind of suffering on the dog because we recognize that the dog is sentient: we feel a duty and obligation to put an end to the torture, and we all agree that Simon's pleasure cannot possibly be a valid reason for inflicting so much suffering on this poor animal.

In the second case of our average American diners, though, most people likely justify the moral wrongs inflicted on animals as "necessary" to feed us. Most of us assume that the animals had to die to nourish us, because we need animal protein to live healthfully. Sure, the reasoning may go, it is a sad state of affairs that other creatures must die to feed us, but such is the way of the world, and being at the top of the food chain, we cannot help but live the way we do. To the extent that someone feels badly about this, they may assuage their consciences by buying "locally raised" meats, or otherwise using products that some giant supermarket chain has convinced them is somehow "humane." But really, nature is red in tooth and claw, the world is this way, and we cannot change it. (One wonders if these people would be angry with the grizzly bear who might eat them during a camping trip, since a passive acceptance of the way things supposedly are with the food chain is such an attractive notion to them.)

But really, do we need to eat meat or animal products to live well? Certainly not! Indeed, a growing body of evidence — much of it backed by long-term epidemiological and clinical studies[2] — would indicate that leaving animal products out of your diet is the more healthful choice. Given this clinically proven fact that we don't need animal products to live healthfully, how then do we justify using them? Most people, including very thoughtful and intelligent people, resort to arguing that "this is the way it has always been," that it is our "culture," our "tradition." Plus, they reason, animal products taste so damn good. But if animal products are not necessary to live healthfully, and if we can easily derive nourishment in ways that do not make animals suffer and die, the question becomes this: in what way does Simon's blowtorching of the dog — or Michael Vick's abuse of pit bulls for sport — become different than our abuse of billions of animals a year for our food? In both cases, neither imposition of suffering is in any way necessary, and both are related to pleasure in the end. Yet, we're horrified by Simon's abuse, and seemingly uninterested in the violence done to bring dairy, eggs, and animal flesh to our plates.

This disconnect between our thoughts and our actions hits at the heart of what Francione considers to be our moral schizophrenia. The average person agrees that we should not inflict unnecessary suffering on animals, yet they'll say so while consuming a hamburger — and they'll often do so without the sense of tragic irony befitting the situation. In the case of Simon torturing the dog, we recognize that the dog has an interest in avoiding suffering because the dog can experience pain. We therefore feel an obligation to end such suffering. We base this not on the dog's intelligence, and not on his ability or inability to communicate in our language, but because we know the dog to be sentient. To be sentient means to be capable of "subjective mental experiences," to have a sense of an "I" who is conscious of pain and pleasure.[3] All sentient beings — humans, primates, cows, pigs, chickens, and rodents — are "similar to each other and dissimilar to everything else in the world that is not sentient."[5] If cows and chickens and dogs are all sentient, and if we agree, at least implicitly, that we should avoid inflicting unnecessary harm on sentient beings, then our infliction of suffering on a chicken destined for our dinner plate merely because we like the taste of chicken is no more valid than Simon inflicting suffering on his dog for the mere pleasure of it.

Animals possess the same elemental neural machinery that we do for experiencing pain and pleasure. For at least the past 200 years, even our laws have recognized that inflicting "unnecessary" suffering on animals should be punished as a criminal matter, and that we should balance our interests in producing animal suffering over the interests of animals to be free of that suffering.[5] The "humane treatment principle" dictates that if no real human interests are at stake, and if we can find alternatives to animal use in a particular situation, we should pursue those alternatives as a matter of principle. However, we tend to approach every animal use as an emergency situation, a "them-or-us" scenario in which we must decide between the interests of animals and humans as a near life-or-death situation. However, as Francione points out, "the overwhelming portion of our animal uses cannot be described as necessary in any meaningful sense of the word; rather, they merely further the satisfaction of human pleasure, amusement, or convenience. This wholly unnecessary animal use results in an enormous amount of animal pain, suffering, and death."[6]

What, then, is the solution to this moral schizophrenia we have about animals? According to Francione, we only have two choices: we either continue to treat animals as we are now, by inflicting suffering even for unnecessary ends and recognizing our commitment to humane treatment as a farce, or, we can recognize that animals have a morally significant interest in not being subjected to unnecessary suffering, and change how we approach conflicts of animal and human interests. To do the latter, however, requires that we apply the principle of equal consideration to animals. This, Francione argues, is stunningly simple: in its most basic terms, we need to treat like cases alike. Though animals and humans are clearly different, they are alike in the sense that they both suffer and are both sentient. For this reason, we should extend the principle of equal consideration to animals.

This means that we should guarantee animals the right not to be treated exclusively as a means to the ends of another, or the right not to be treated as things. Animals, however, are mere things today, the property of their owners and — at least legally — not much more. Animals "belong" to people, or legal people like corporations, in much the same way that any other piece of property does. The farmer can sell and buy cows; the vivisector can purchase mice prone to develop certain kinds of diseases; you and I can buy purebred designer dogs or cats if we wish. To many of us, this seems like an everyday fact of life. We are so accustomed to thinking of animals as our property that we rarely think of the impacts of this legal and social status for animals. For example, were we fickle pet owners and were we to tire of living with the dog who is always sleeping near one of us as we write, we could sell her for whatever we felt was a fair price. Emmy (our dog) is our legal property. Were she worth enough, we could leverage her as collateral for a debt. Similarly, if someone came along and wanted to pay $500 for her, we could certainly and legally sell her for that price. Though we shudder to even say such a thing, we could take her to the vet right now and have her euthanized if we wished. In either case, because she is our property, we are more or less free to dispose of her as we wish. She is, in every way, at our mercy since she is ours in every conceivable way.

With farm animals, the same thing applies. Take, for example, the chickens who spend their entire lives jammed up in tiny cages or overcrowded "cage-free" coops laying eggs. Once they are finished providing profit for their owners, they are often gassed or slaughtered *en masse*, since they are now no longer worth anything. They're living beings, but they lack any recourse to life, because the person who owns them has decided otherwise. This power of ownership does not begin at slaughter; from just about the moment the chicken is conceived, owners can leverage control, turning an animal into a living machine for profit. As such, the owner of the hen has the right under the law to treat the hen almost as he wishes; he can starve the hen for a forced molt to increase productivity; he can imprison the hen in a tiny cage with six or seven other hens; and, after the hen has ceased being useful property, he can dispose of the hen by gassing her or breaking her neck. The point here is that the hen serves as little more than the means to the end of producing eggs, and thus producing profit for the owner. This makes the hen exclusively the means of another, and turns her into a thing, a mere commodity. None of us would ever wish to be the mere instrument of another, to have our entire being tied up in the profit motives and wishes of another. Yet, we routinely live our lives in ways that keep this vicious process going on and on.

In working through the implications of living things being merely property, Francione emphasizes that we used to have humans that were also mere means to the ends of another: we called them slaves, and human slavery functioned in much the same way as animal slavery does. We abolished human slavery because we recognized long ago that all humans have intrinsic and inherent value beyond their ability to serve as a resource to others. For Francione, inherent value is:

> *merely another name for the minimal criterion necessary*
> *to be regarded as a member of the moral community. If*
> *you do not have inherent value, all of your interests —*
> *including your fundamental interest in not experiencing*
> *pain and your interest in continued life — can be "sold*
> *away," depending on someone else's valuation. In order*
> *for the concept of inherent value to protect humans from*
> *being treated as things, we must regard all humans as*
> *having equal inherent value.*[7]

The notion of equal inherent value applies even if a human is, say, mentally incapacitated: few of us would ever agree that we could use a severely mentally disabled person for medical experiments. Why? Because there's something chillingly wrong with the idea — it feels monstrous, and harkens back to the darkest periods of modern history when Nazi doctors routinely used human beings as lab animals. To put it more directly, we feel sick because we recognize and respect the inherent value of the mentally incapacitated person not to be the end of another. This basic right not to be treated as a thing is, Francione illustrates, the minimum necessary requirement for membership in the moral community. Extremely basic, but totally essential, this basic right not to be turned into a mere thing, a piece of property without interests, is something that we afford even the least among us as human beings. All of us expect and demand this for ourselves, and we hopefully expect and demand this for others. Moreover, we also all know and understand that even humans who lack what we consider rationality or self-awareness enjoy this same basic right. Very young infants are neither rational nor meaningfully self-aware, yet we extend them the basic right not to be treated as things. Clearly, an infant has a very different set of capacities than a full-grown adult. We don't (nor should we) grant infants every possible right that a full-grown adult has. It probably wouldn't do most infants much good to have the right to vote, drive, or enter into contracts. Yet, no one in her right mind suggests that experimenting on human infants is acceptable simply because at a certain young age, they lack rationality or language or the ability to notice their own reflection in a mirror, all because we grant them this stunningly simple yet vitally important right: namely, that they cannot be treated simply as the ends of another.

Expanding Equal Consideration

Much as humanity has extended this basic equal consideration to humans (including those who were once considered to be less-than-human, or outside of our moral community), we must extend this basic equal consideration to animals if we are going to treat like cases alike. Animals are very clearly in possession of a subjective experience of their own lives. Anyone who lives with companion animals knows this to be true. We live with two dogs and three cats, and each of them has wants, moods, desires, and needs. They are not mere automatons, reacting machine-like to the stimuli around them. Instead, they are beings that are aware of themselves, their environment, and those around them. Our dogs communicate with us; Emmy will often run to where her leash is, staring up, and barking if she wants to go out. Mole will often come and drop toys in our lap when he wants to play. Our little kitty Spike will sometimes bring in the crumpled up paper balls we chuck at him when he wants to bat them around on the floor for a while. We live our lives with these animals, and we know them to be more than simple things. Like any of us, they seek out pleasure and affection and avoid pain, and it is entirely clear that they have a subjective mental life. We can argue about their intelligence (which we would likely define in human-centric terms anyway), their ability to understand human language, or even the extent to which they really understand and know the world around them, but there's no argument that can convincingly show that animals don't feel pain, and that they have no interest in avoiding that pain. If anything, animals are more sensitive to the world around them than we are, given their heightened sensory abilities.

Though we use the example of the dogs with whom we live, Bob has also been around enough animals who are involved in agricultural production to know that they are also capable of forming bonds with others and with humans, and that they, too, are capable of feeling pain and pleasure. We obviously don't believe that every animal in the world is like our cats and dogs. Instead, we're simply looking at things logically, and working them through to their ethical conclusions. If we're going to be consistent about how we treat cases that are alike, we ought to recognize the fact that animals have as much an interest in avoiding suffering as we do. "In the case of animals," Francione writes "the principle of equal consideration tells us that if we are going to take animal interests seriously and give content to the prohibition against unnecessary suffering that we all claim to accept, then we must extend the same protection to animal interests in not suffering unless we have a good reason for doing so."[8]

Note that neither our taste, nor our convenience, desire, culture, nor tradition constitute a "good reason" here. Because animals clearly are sentient and because they suffer, they deserve inclusion in our ethical community. If we can end this particularly bloody and violent form of slavery, there seems to be little reason to continue doing it, apart from our mere tastes and customs. As with any societal privilege, many of us directly benefit from this particular form of oppression. Many people enjoy their leather jackets, their "happy meat" from Whole Foods, and their unpasteurized European cheeses. Yet, these products, and any other animal products, are sullied by a long history in which animals are dominated for our wants, tastes, and pleasures — and nothing more. Because of this almost unilateral benefit that many of us accrue by virtue of our species, we are by and large unwilling to see how this oppression affects the animal "other."

People who do work educating whites about white privilege and structural racism run into the same phenomenon. Those who benefit from whiteness, or patriarchy, or class, or any of the other social structures that ensure the reproduction of privilege in our world often fail to see how they are privileged; it is so thoroughly taken for granted that it is like trying to explain water to a fish. Similarly, our dominance as humans is so taken for granted that explaining our species privilege — even to people who profess to be deeply concerned about social justice causes of all stripes — is quite difficult. Nevertheless, these are relations of economic and social power that we are participating in. The fact that we can confine and kill animals for our ends (even incredibly frivolous ones) speaks a great deal about the hierarchy that we exercise both over animals and the rest of the natural world. By compelling animals to produce for us, we (knowingly or unknowingly) take part in maintaining the domination of humanity over the natural world and its inhabitants, and such exploitation is often justified with stunningly simplistic logic. People who otherwise spend their time concerned about equity and justice will often argue that animals are "here for us" to consume, that our might makes right, and that there is really no other choice if we want to eat. Such logic only serves to prop up an exploitative and violent system of dominance, much as every other exploitative system of dominance and hierarchy that humanity has dealt with over the ages.

The Importance of Consistency

In so far as animals are like us, they deserve rights like ours. In practical terms, this means that they deserve to live in a way that comports with their nature and instincts, and to be something other than property. Animals need to be ends in themselves and for themselves, and not just the means to our ends. For this inherent value to be realized, animals have to no longer be the property of another. Until then, animals will be subject to unimaginable suffering, since property can never have interests that are more important than those of the property owner.

Veganism is the single most powerful way of rejecting this propertied relationship in your own life, but on its own, it is not enough. Your veganism must be part of a larger movement of activism and outreach that functions such that we do not continue to remake or uphold the property relationship as it applies to animals. For this reason, we urge you to rely on vegan education as the defining character of your activism. The further afield we go from our base in veganism, the weaker and more contradictory the message can become.

Along these lines, we have two points to make on the vital importance of consistency.

First, if you want to make an impact in the lives of animals, don't bother negotiating for bigger cages, or nicer accommodations, or more humane slaughter methods. Instead, cut right to the heart of the matter, and get as many people as you can to go vegan. At first glance, this advice about not negotiating for bigger cages and the like might seem contradictory. Why, you might ask, would we object to people working to make conditions better for animals who are certainly suffering? Obviously, less suffering is preferable to more suffering, and there are a great many compelling reasons to want animals to suffer less. Yet, many of the measures that are designed to improve animal welfare standards actually end up helping the industries that exploit animals to sell more animal products. Remember: the kinds of activism we pursue matter, and their relationship with our overall goals is essential. We want a world that's free of animal exploitation, not one in which nicer forms become more acceptable. On top of this, many of these so-called "reforms" actually just end up making people who might otherwise object to animal agriculture feel more comfortable with the meat they're eating. The pangs of guilt that the conscientious feel are assuaged by labels like "free range," "local," "organic," and "humane," but all these labels do is guarantee that a tiny percentage of animals live a life that is somewhat less hellish. By failing to effectively counter the demand for animal products, this kind of activism also does nothing to fight the problem at its source, leaving in place the same, old ugly dynamics that led to the killing in the first place.

The justifications for this kind of "activism" are many, but none are compelling. People will tell you that we can't change the way people eat, and so we have to take what we can get. Others will say that this will lead to some kind of vast incremental change over time in which we will garner more rights for animals as we progress. Yet others will say that this is all we can hope to ask for, and if we ask for too much, we'll get nothing. It is all bullshit. It might be well-meaning bullshit, but it is bullshit nevertheless. If we believe that we can't change the way people see things, we've accepted defeat before we've even begun. If incremental change is coming, where is it, and why are more animals being killed every year than the year before? If we're going to fight for the rights of

animals, how are we going to do so while we're simultaneously helping industries that exploit them and kill them make
a more marketable product?

If you still might not be getting the point of our criticism, think
of it this way: imagine that a horrible genocide is taking place
in which millions of people are being killed mercilessly for
absolutely no reason. Children and being taken from their
mothers at birth, and adults are forced to labor for a time, and
then violently murdered by being hacked apart by machetes
when they are no longer useful. Enraged by the genocide, a
large, multimillion-dollar human rights organization begins a
huge campaign designed to change the policies of the government committing the genocide. Publicly, the organization says
that they are opposed to the killing, and that they abhor and
want to abolish genocide. But despite this policy, the organization works closely with the genocidal government so that
every person killed in the genocide is gently put to sleep
with a cocktail of powerful chemicals instead of being hacked
apart by knives. As a result of the new policy, however, the
genocidal regime is able to be even more efficient in its killing,
since this new kind of chemical murder requires less labor.

Hopefully, the absurdity of this position is obvious to you. In
this situation, the organization that works with the genocidal
regime is complicit. Sure, at one level, they're objecting to the
horrendousness of it all. But at another level, they're completely missing the point. While there's no doubt that dying in
a way that's like a nap is preferable to dying in storm of
machete hacks, *the real problem is that people are being killed.*
The genocide needs to stop; it doesn't need to be done more
nicely. No human rights organization that we know of would
articulate such a ridiculous position, but almost every animal
rights organization we've encountered routinely advocates an
equivalent for animals. To us, this isn't innovative activism

that deals with the realities of the world. It is, plain and simple, nothing but damning more and more animals to lives of total misery because people will be led to believe that what they're eating is somehow more kind and less cruel. The inherent worth of animals isn't recognized, animals remain property, and they are still killed and eaten by the billions, all while just about every animal rights organization pumps a near-endless supply of dollars into measures that help the industries that exploit animals sell more product, because now it can be marketed as somehow less cruel.

Activism like this is odd for any vegan to pursue. If you do it, you'll see that before long, you'll be making arguments for the consumption of one kind of animal product over another, and it gets to be a bit like making advocating for one kind of genocidal death over another. Though neither of us have been part of any human rights organization that failed to take an effective stance against genocide, Bob was briefly involved in a campaign organized and funded by a large animal rights organization, and that involvement was what got us both thinking about what our activism meant, and how we needed to be consistent in our approach. A number of years ago, back when we were college professors, Bob was working with a fledgling animal rights group on the campus of the University where we worked, mostly helping to get the group off the ground, and serving as a kind of advisor, contact point, and resource. Wanting to get involved in some local activism, the group decided that they were interested in getting the University to use all cage-free eggs in their dining facilities, as opposed to eggs that came from hens confined to cages. With no small amount of gusto, the group began this campaign, working to educate people about the differences between the eggs, and leaning on the University administration to make the switch. In preparation for a meeting with the dining services staff, Bob had to call up a few cage-free egg operations recommended to him by this certain large organization. Information in hand, Bob ended up passing on important details about shelf life and shipping time to the University. But in doing so, he had the sudden realization that as a vegan, he was actually helping to make an argument that one animal product was better than another, and that this in and of itself was an argument whose premise was, for lack of a better term, totally fucked.

Bob was a vegan then and is a vegan now. Bob was also pretty freaked out when he realized that as a vegan, he was actually urging people to eat eggs. The point of veganism isn't to encourage people to eat eggs that are raised in what are allegedly better conditions — the point of veganism is *to get people not to eat any goddamn eggs at all, from any source, anywhere!* The argument to make to people isn't one about which animal product is more humane or more happy — the argument to make is that animal products are laced with incredible cruelty, and that any of them mean that an animal somewhere was subjugated to make the product for you. The argument is that we can live without these things, not that we need to find more allegedly "humane" ways to make them. Only by doing this can we get people to go vegan, which is the only thing that effectively attacks the roots of the problem.

Second, if we are opposed to the violence done to animals, we must oppose violence in our activism and outreach. We know that we'll be called collaborators, tools of the state, traitors, informants, and a thousand other dirty things because we make this point, but we don't care. The point is important, and it needs to be made. Put in the most stark terms possible, there's no way to logically argue that violence against animals is wrong while simultaneously engaging in violence yourself. By violence, we envision the obvious things that entail hurting other beings, but we also take property destruction, threats, and intimidation to be forms of violence, because they impact people in ways that are remarkably like the impacts of physical violence. We get that what is being done to animals is rage inducing. We understand the helplessness and frustration that you might feel. But the way to combat these feelings is by helping to build a genuine movement of vegans, not by destroying something and re-creating the dynamic of power and force that we all supposedly detest so much.

Apart from the ethical contradictions of violence for a movement that is intrinsically non-violent, there are practical considerations that make violence pointless for the cause of animal rights. First, something like 99 percent of the population believes that eating animals is just fine. In the context of a culture like this, how does violent action make any sense at all? No one understands what it is for, it has an extremely limited impact, and the full repressive machinery of the state is not only hauled out to keep activists in check, it is cheered on by the majority of people who have absolutely no frame of reference for understanding why any violent action was done in the first place.

Second, as the authors of an old anarchist pamphlet said long ago, "you can't blow up a social relationship." By this they mean that the way society is organized is something that runs so deep within us that blowing stuff up accomplishes nothing because it does not help people to understand what is wrong in the first place. The only way that we will ever unravel this sociopathic system that condemns animals to lives of utter misery is by doing the hard work of getting people to see that the social relationship between animals and humans is broken in fundamental ways. Blowing up slaughterhouses or vivisection labs or whatever the target du jour is for the misanthropic movement tourists who like blowing shit up won't accomplish a thing towards this end, and it may, in fact, cement feelings in the complete opposite direction through a widespread public backlash.

We've said it many times, and we'll say it many more times: the only effective solution is to embrace non-violent vegan activism that works to reach people in their everyday lives. As vegans, we can promote incredible change, but to do that, we have to believe in ourselves and in the essential power of our message. Veganism means living your activism, and living it in ways that fit with the underlying principles that veganism espouses.

Veganism is Living Your Activism

Sadly, a great many are unwilling to take up the struggle, but animal exploitation is undeniably an imposition of the will of the strong on the weak. Veganism and non-violent vegan activism and education are the primary vehicles for effectively combating this imposition of will and this stark social injustice. The only way we can ever effectively overcome the exploitative dominance that humans have over animals is to change society, and this requires building a movement of people who are working conscientiously and nonviolently to educate people around them about the importance of veganism. Were there any fantastic shortcuts to the kind of world we were after, people much smarter than us would have figured them out long ago. The bad news here is that this leaves us all with the hard work of changing things where the odds are overwhelming against us. The good news is that the tools that we need are ones we already have: ourselves, our talents, and our energies.

Forget the Organizations: Empower Yourself

Though there is certainly some active, inventive, and creative grassroots activism going on in the animal rights community, there is a pervasive notion that we should leave the most important activism to the "professionals." Yet, this idea is horribly pernicious. As the large, multi-million dollar animal advocacy organizations have become gradually co-opted in a familiar process of give and take with industry they claim to oppose, they become less and less able to effectively combat animal exploitation at its roots.

Because these organizations must rely on "winnable" campaigns and donations to stay alive, they are limited not only in the scope of actions they can take, but also in the kinds of campaigns they can support. As they become more co-opted, the movement organizations gradually become more and more conservative, even if they don themselves in the mask of radicalism — something at which PETA is particularly adept. A more conservative outlook is a pragmatic matter of institutional survival, and while it is useful for keeping the organizations alive and maintaining their bureaucracies, it also has ripple effects throughout the animal rights movement. As the giants of the movement, these organizations have the power to define agendas, garner media attention, and influence the terms upon which debate will be carried out. Most people who care about animals and are otherwise not involved in the animal rights movement end up seeing their concern channeled and focused by these larger organizations, and that concern is channeled in ways that actually end up doing little to effectively combat animal exploitation. Simultaneously, the kinds of participation that larger organizations encourage also leads to a more widespread disempowerment when it comes to animal rights activism.

These dynamics are most apparent in the reliance on money and memberships. If you're unlucky enough to have your name end up on some of the mailing lists that we happen to be on, you will receive a deluge of junk mail from animal rights organizations, every single piece of which begs for money in some way or another. Borrowing from the worst marketing practices of corporations, some of these pieces of junk mail even request participation in a "survey," yet the survey itself is merely a psychological marketing ploy, designed to remind people of the horrors of animal exploitation before the pitch for cash at the end of the letter. Almost all of the appeals for "memberships" promise that YOU can do something for animals — if only you'll give the organization in question just $25, $50, $100, or even $500 of your money.

Recycle the offers, and keep your money. Instead of sending it to PETA or the Humane Society or whomever, use your cash to organize something locally so you can educate people about the importance of veganism. You'll get a much better bang for your buck or yen or pound or euro or whatever, and you'll know exactly what the money is going towards. For next to nothing, or even for free, you can get the word out. Show a film that highlights the problems of animal exploitation, and gets people thinking. Host a discussion at your local library. Start an animal rights reading group with friends. Bring a speaker to your campus. Have a vegan potluck. Make up some pamphlets and give them out. Make art that gets people to think about the situation of animals. Write books and pamphlets to help people see the importance of this issue. Give away vegan food. Cook something for your friends and family that's vegan, and remind them that it is. The number of things that you can do is limited only by your imagination, and the only way we will ever make any real change in the world is to begin doing it ourselves. Find people who share your vision and goals on these important issues, and get out into the world and use your talents to draw attention to these vitally important issues. Alone or in a small group of friends, you have the ability to reach people that no organization can, large or small. You know how the people around you think, and you can tailor messages and forms of activism that can speak to people in ways they understand and are sympathetic to. You have the ability to communicate this message to people, and to help grow this movement. No one else — not PETA or the Humane Society or any other big group — can be nearly as powerful as you can be if you are a thoughtful, hard-working, and non-violent activist in your daily life.

Granted, it is easier to send money to the big organizations, but if we're going to ever change anything, we need you to be more than a check-writer for the big organizations. We know that what we propose is slippery and ambiguous — we're asking you to think, to rely on yourself and your wits, and to give of yourself in ways that no organization would ever ask. Yes, you'll have to figure some things out on your own, but that's the beauty of it. Not only can you help to bring about an important change in the way that people see things, you can also help to fight the sinking feeling of anger, frustration, and helplessness that often goes along with the knowledge that you have about the horrible situation animals are in. The best antidote to despair is action. Writing a check to PETA so they can buy another chicken costume, or put another naked star on some billboard, or advertise the award they've given to a slaughterhouse designer[9] might feel good for a day or two after you've put the check in the mail, but the glow fades fast. Nothing is nearly as powerful as you taking ownership of your own activism.

IN THIS CHAPTER AND THROUGHOUT THIS BOOK, our emphasis is on veganism as the lived expression of the abolitionist approach to animal rights. Veganism is and always has been about animal rights, and we hope that it will continue to serve as a powerful intervention in the incredibly troubled relationship that humans have with animals. Still, we must touch on two final points before we close out the chapter, which will at least provide you with some food for thought as you move into your own veganism and/or vegan activism.

Enviro-veganism

If you start doing even the most casual kind of research on intensive animal agriculture, you quickly discover that there are a handful of what appear to be very compelling reasons to go vegan on account of the environment. Whether you're repulsed by the lagoons of manure that people sometimes drown in, or the idea that raising cattle creates more greenhouse gas than driving, environmental concerns do certainly compel some people to go vegan, and that's a good thing.

Yet, going vegan solely for environmental reasons is a fundamental misunderstanding of what veganism is at its very roots. With ecosexualism at an all-time high these days, and the so-called "green" movement having its own cable channel in the US and a whole range of "green" products to consume, we'd be swimming against a strong tide to suggest that anything done for environmental reasons is somehow not something done for a good reason. Truth is, we're grateful for the bourgeoning number of envirovegans out there. If the environment gets people thinking about veganism and moving towards veganism, that's a good thing indeed, but ultimately, veganism is about the inherent personhood of animals, and at its core, it has one fundamental goal: recognizing the rights of non-humans.

Since the very day the term "vegan" was coined by Donald and Dot Watson back the 1940s, veganism has been about the rights of non-humans to receive equal consideration. Veganism has evolved in some very strange ways indeed, but today, full-fledged veganism is still the only rational response that hits at the roots of animal exploitation. As we've said innumerable times in these pages, veganism is your everyday statement that things are not right as they are, your standing up and being counted as one more person opposed to the bloody machinery of animal agriculture. Veganism is about animal rights.

So, while we're grateful for all of the environmental vegans out there, a mere environmental impetus all by itself is an inadequate foundation for a long-term vegan perspective, or for really founding a long-term movement that seeks to accord animals substantial rights. To put it another way, going vegan for mere environmental reasons is rather like opposing the Holocaust because the trains to Auschwitz had a large carbon footprint. Now, before you get your under-garments all bunched up in your crack and get all morally indignant and righteous on us, stop, take a deep breath, and think about the essential point we're making. In either case, the person is opposed to the Holocaust. But most of us would argue that the person objecting on environmental grounds is rather missing the larger point here: namely, that genocide is deeply repulsive and horribly wrong because it violates the basic rights that we think all human beings should have. The worry that the trains are belching carbon into the sky seems disconnected, and honestly, a bit sick.

With tens of billions of animals dying around the world each year, we're looking at a situation that is, by all accounts, horrible for the environment. There's no doubt that this par-ticular form of killing is strangling ecosystems. But being vegan mostly or solely for environmental reasons misses the point of veganism. For ethical vegans, the point of veganism is to recognize the inherent value of animals as beings in their own right. Though the environmental side effects of the exploitation of humans and non-humans alike are drastic, worrying, and taking an ever-greater toll on our ecosystems, we nevertheless have to put these concerns within a larger context of exploitation, one in which the environmental side effects of exploitation are understood, but not in which they're the central aspect of our concern.

Fuck the Body Politics Already

Authors far craftier than us have sold millions of books by convincing women that going vegan is a fantastic way to squeeze into that hot little black "fuck me" dress.

Well, fuck that.

These kinds of body politics are pernicious. They suggest to women that in order to be beautiful, they must conform to a standard of beauty that is often dangerous or impossible to achieve. The unspoken threat hanging out there is that if you don't get skinny, that you'll be ugly, unloved, and miserable. And then, *omigod,* you'll never attract a man worth having if you're all fat and plump and shit. (If you ever wondered if sexism was still alive and well, there's your proof.)

No doubt, the hope of skinny is foreclosed for women who are unfortunate enough to be born with hips and boobs. Skinny, apparently, means looking like a teenage boy who suffered through a famine. Maybe it is just Bob being Latino, but come on — booty is a beautiful thing! People come in all different sizes and shapes and colors, and we can't all look like Gwyneth Fucking Paltrow or whomever happens to be hot this week. There's no reason that anyone should hate themselves because they feel fat, or because they were so cursed as to be born with ... Dare we say it? ... *curves!*

As a movement that fights exploitation and oppression, we should refuse to be exploitative and oppressive. We can't legitimately use arguments that oppress and exploit women through ridiculous and unachievable notions of beauty and body size to argue that we should not be exploiting another group that is vulnerable to deep and pervasive social injustice. We must demand more of ourselves as activists and thinkers, and look towards better ways of treating one another, ways that build each other up and welcome people, rather than tearing people down. Oprah's cleanse is misleading, and so is the notion that veganism is a starvation diet that can make you can look more "bangable" to people who are shallow enough to give a shit how much you weigh. The abolitionist vegan movement we're trying to grow by our work here is one that should be inclusive. Whether you're big or small, able-bodied or disabled, straight or gay or bi, or male or female or whatever other gender expression you make your own, you'll have a place here. We don't care if you're skinny, and we don't care if you're a bitch. We only care that you're helping others to see why this ridiculous exploitation of animals has to stop.

BY LIVING AS A VEGAN, you are making a stand, and living in the world as you would like to see it — free of animal exploitation. Veganism goes beyond what we put in our mouths and wear on our bodies; it is a statement against our moral schizophrenia towards animals that pervades our society. Veganism is a stand against the status of animals as property. It is also a direct intervention that stands against the exploitation of sentient beings that deserve equal consideration in our moral community. Since we were only able to provide an introduction to these concepts and the abolitionist approach to animal rights in this chapter, we repeat our recommendation from earlier, and urge you to check out Gary Francione's book *Introduction to Animal Rights: Your Child or the Dog*, an indispensable guide to understanding rights theory, as well as Bob's book *Making a Killing: The Political Economy of Animal Rights*, an analysis of animals as commodities and property in our modern capitalist society. Both books will help you to learn more about the arguments and logic presented here.

IF YOU CAN FORGIVE US for failing to solve the North Korea Problem despite what looks like our declarations to the contrary, you will hopefully be walking away from this chapter secure in your choice to go vegan. We don't need to tell you yet again how important it is to go vegan, so we won't. But we will say that going vegan is pretty damn easy, though there are usually some small things to deal with along the way, particularly as the choice to go vegan starts bumping up the everyday confines of your own situation. In the coming chapters, we get down into the nitty-gritty, nuts-and-bolts kinds of things, like figuring out how to deal with the people in your life and figuring out what to eat and buy so that you can live your ethics as consistently as possible. Even if you're still on the fence because you think it is too difficult to be vegan, these chapters will show you that it's really not that hard once you get the hang of a few key things, and before you know it, you'll be a pompous, fun-killing, food-hating, radical-extremist vegan just like the rest of us.

Notes to Chapter 2

1   Much of this chapter is adapted from Bob's book *Making a Killing: The Political Economy of Animal Rights*, which addresses these topics and themes in much greater detail than is necessary here.

2   For a good overview of many of the studies on this point and compelling original research, see also T. Colin Campbell and Thomas M. Campbell II, *The China Study: The Most Comprehensive Study of Nutrition Ever Conducted and the Startling Implications for Diet, Weight Loss, and Long-Term Health* (Dallas: Benbella Books, 2006).

3   Francione, *Introduction to Animal Rights: Your Child or the Dog?*, 6.

4   Ibid.

5   Francione, *Introduction to Animal Rights: Your Child or the Dog?*, 8-9.

6   Ibid., 9.

7   Ibid., 96.

8   Ibid., 99.

9   People for the Ethical Treatment of Animas (PETA), 2004 Peta Proggy Awards, http://peta.org/feat/proggy/2004/index.html.

CHAPTER 3

HELL IS OTHER PEOPLE

IN THE FIRST VERSION OF THIS BOOK, we told the story of Bob's Uncle Bill. In case you never heard about Uncle Bill (or UB as we often call him) from us on our podcast, he's your typical dirty uncle — he's politically incorrect, he loves to forward the millions of dirty jokes he gets over email, and he has a world-class appreciation for toilet humor. He still smokes, still eats fast food (especially when he can get coupons for a good deal), and pretty much does and says whatever he wants, especially if it will get a rise out of someone.

When we first became vegan, we sat down next to Uncle Bill at Christmas dinner, and managed to work our way through the entire meal without any comments about the fact that the turkey was missing from our plates and that we had special mashed potatoes and stuffing set aside for us. As dinner ended, we sat back, thinking we were in the clear. No rude comments from UB? How could it be? Was Christmas turning the guy into a softie or something?

Apparently, it was too good to be true. Sitting back in our chairs enjoying our relative holiday success with a warm mug of coffee with soymilk, Uncle Bill sidled up to the table, eyed up the soymilk carton, and made a face.

Aww shit, here it comes.

UB, the great Archie Bunker of Philadelphia, gave the soymilk a once-over. As the very idea of soymilk found its way into one of the cracks in his brain between all the dirty jokes and bawdy stories, you could see his expression change from a smirk to utter disgust. Putting the carton down as though it was a plague-riddled rat ready to bite him, UB said, "I'd rather enjoy what I eat than die young than drink this shit. All this healthy crap out there... who the hell wants it? You don't really like this shit, do you?"

At this point, the one thing you have to realize is that Bob isn't the kind of guy to run from an argument. In fact, some sick little part of him enjoys annoying people for sport, which is why so many people over the years have told him he'd make a great lawyer. Having had the "enemy" engage, Bob seemed ready to pounce. Actually, if Jenna was right, Bob was looking forward to pouncing.

"Yeah, we drink it. You should try it, it is pretty good," Bob replied in a friendly tone. Truth be told, Bob surprised even himself with this move. In the past, Bob would have hunkered down for a fight whenever anyone challenged him — and maybe even if they didn't. Bob is a real bastard if you cross him, and he never lets up. But somehow, on this day, Bob had matured beyond the skate punk "fuck off" ethos, at least for the moment. And most surprisingly, it worked.

"Yeah, well, I'd never try that stuff," UB said, putting down the carton. Then he walked away.

That's right. He walked away! No more jokes. No more teasing. No more stupid cuts on vegans — nothing. By not getting upset over a stupid crack about soymilk, Bob denied UB the chance to get a rise out of us, something which he would have

enjoyed immensely. Since he tried and got nowhere with us, the game lost its appeal, and he immediately sensed there'd be no point in pushing it much further, particularly with so many offensive blonde jokes waiting in the wings.

Since that Christmas a few years back, we've seen Uncle Bill on many holidays and the occasional Sunday dinner, and he always makes some crack about what we are eating.

"Is this the vegan stuff? No way I'm eating that shit."

"Can you pass the creamer? The real stuff, not that soy crap."

"Hey, I'm feeling constipated. Can I try some of that vegan food so I can take a nice huge shit tomorrow?"

"What the hell is that made with anyway?"

Through the years, we've been good about letting the comments slide and just chuckling about them. (The lone exception is the one time UB was dumb enough to say something rude about how the Christmas cookies Jenna had spent days making were shit because they were vegan. Bob thought for a split second that Jenna was going to jump across the table and punch him, but somehow, she held back.)

After six years of making cracks about vegan food, something amazing happened, and not even we could believe it. Yes, after six years, Bill actually came out and admitted one night that he "kind of liked some of that vegan shit." We were stunned, nonplussed, gobsmacked — whatever you want to call it, it was a moment of utter surprise. Sure, we already knew UB was fine with at least some vegan food since we often have to keep Bill from eating some of that "weird vegan shit" at family dinners before we can get a chance to try it, but this time, he actually seemed to be admitting to himself that he liked something vegan. He said it out loud, and he wasn't joking! Granted, it took years, but the moral of the story is that with patience and the right attitude, even the most die-hard veganophobe can come around, even if only a little. And in this game, you have to take your victories where you can get them, no matter how small they may seem.

Sad as it is, the world is not always a vegan-friendly place, and Uncle Bill is but one example of the kinds of people you'll have to deal with as a vegan. Although it is not difficult to be vegan once you get the hang of things, you're going to have to deal with many non-vegan situations (such as dinner at Aunt Edna's) and interact with a lot of non-vegan people (in all likelihood, just about everyone you know). After a few weeks of stupid questions, taunts, and general misunderstanding of why you are doing what you are doing, you may feel tempted to go out and start your own vegan commune somewhere. Tempting though it may be, that is neither necessary nor desirable — how can we make the world more vegan-friendly if we're off hiding somewhere by ourselves? — since there are ways to mitigate the pain of interacting with people who just don't get it. In this chapter, we'll give you advice on staying sane, true to yourself and proud of your veganism in the face of this insane world of ours. However, before we dive into the specifics on how exactly to deal with other people, we first want to talk a little about why it is that people will get so upset, angry, or confused in reaction to you, and why it doesn't make sense to flip out on them.

The Mind of a Meat Eater

Once you've made the decision to go vegan, figuring out what to eat will most likely be the easiest part. It's dealing with the non-vegans in your life that presents the most challenges, generates the most dread, and provides the most friction. After all, we're social creatures. We go out to eat with our friends, we make small talk with our co-workers, and we celebrate holidays with our families. As a vegan, however, your relationship to all of these people inevitably changes, even if you're the exact same person in every other realm of your life. By being a vegan, you're rejecting something that they think is completely normal and acceptable, and every time you put a fork in your mouth, you remind them of that fact.

Most people are simply not ready to hear the truth about their food just yet — particularly while they are eating. Sure, in an abstract way they know that meat comes from animals, but they don't want to know that veal calves are tortured and left in the dark from almost their first day on the face of the earth, or that layer hens are stacked seven to a tiny cage for their entire lives. As consumers, we possess impressive repressive machinery that has its roots in the way that we're raised in capitalist, Western culture. Meat eaters or not, we generally don't think much about where anything we produce comes from. Those who produce what we consume generally toil away in horrid conditions (and the more horrid the conditions, the lower the price) to make cheap shit we can buy at Wal-Mart. Our cheap sneakers come at the cost of exploiting labor somewhere down the line. Similarly, our cheap meat, eggs, and dairy come not only from exploiting animals, but also exploiting and dehumanizing the people that are involved in the production of these commodities. Just as we "innocently" presume that the person who made our cheap sneakers is being paid fairly for their work we often "innocently" presume that animal agriculture operates with the welfare of animals and workers in mind. From the previous chapters, we know it doesn't. In both cases, there are examples where there's more rather than less justice for the oppressed and exploited, but these examples are far and few between.

More often than not, horrid, barbaric things are done to make a few extra dollars, and unfortunately, there's no shortage of people ready to exploit animals — human and non-human — for a few pennies more profit. Sadly, most of us are ready to buy what they produce. And of course, there's a related question of whether ignorance truly is bliss, or even a valid excuse.

The point here is that in capitalist cultures, we're acculturated to see only things and not to see the relationships that went into producing those things. This applies to our food as readily as it does to any other product. As a vegan, you complicate this relationship by reminding people that there's something wrong at the heart of the matter when it comes to animals. Having seen beyond the pale of the product, having peered into the other side of suffering, exploitation, and death, we know meat is dead, and every sip of milk and every bite of egg contains within it suffering beyond words. To us, these products look dead, and for many vegans they arouse disgust and even nausea.

The problem is that we possess information that everyone else doesn't have, or doesn't want to think about. Knowing what we know, we want to tell everyone, because many of us are convinced that if people knew the truth, they might stop the bloodbath. To vegans, veal is nothing but pointless abuse and murder. To others, it's a delicacy, and this is where things get tough. When you breach this wall that separates meat eating from meat, you're breaching years and years of active repression of this knowledge. In addition to the repressive machinery we described above that comes from not seeing all that goes into production in a capitalist society, we as humans also possess an impressive psychological repressive machinery that deals with the pain of learning the truth about horrific acts. Even when one learns about what really happens in animal agriculture, chances are that the information gets shunted into the back of our minds or is barely processed so that we can go about our daily business of eating animals and using products produced under oppressive conditions without feeling guilty or depressed. Most people's brains just don't want to or can't deal with the information, and most people just don't have it in them to go against the grain. Acknowledging what is really going on means that people either have to come to terms with the truth and do something about it, or they have to live with themselves if they don't do something about it. Either way, the easiest thing is to not think about it at all and just keep up the status quo.

Most meat eaters would prefer to be "innocent" consumers, but intentionally or otherwise, we're there reminding them that they are not, and cannot be. Just by being vegan at a table with non-vegans, even without opening our mouths, we make the uncomfortable truth where meat comes from come to the surface. Carol Adams explains in her book *The Pornography of Meat* that when you practice veganism, you're essentially "standing in" for the animal who's now a thing (food) and no longer present. This makes many non-vegans feel at the very least uncomfortable and a little guilty, and at the most angry and defensive. In fact, if people do get extremely defensive around you (again, even without having said a word about what they're eating), chances are you've hit a nerve with them. The connection between the meat and the sentient being it once was is in the back of their minds somewhere, and you are the reminder that there is something not quite right with how the meat got to the table.

In addition to all of this, you also need to remember that food isn't just what we eat to give us energy and keep us alive. As we said in Chapter 1, food is a powerful social marker — what we eat often tells us about who we are. Chances are, there are at least one or two dishes that your grandparents passed down to your parents that have special meaning for your family for some reason or another — it's what people in their neighborhood ate, it's what people in their ethnic group ate, it's what people in their family ate, it's what people in their region ate — it's what people like them ate. By giving up foods that are part of these traditions, you're often going to be seen as rejecting your family or your upbringing, not the cruelty often inherent in the traditions. In fact, as we mention in the section on family, most people just don't understand that we would love to have the same old dishes we've always had — just in a form where no one had to die to create them.

As you can see, food is fraught with emotional, psychological, and cultural significance. We eat not just to satisfy a physiological hunger, but also to satisfy our emotional needs, to celebrate, to connect with our families, and to mark where we come from. It's no wonder, then, that other people get quite agitated when you are seen as upsetting the balance of these systems, and why they often don't really understand the point of veganism. Most people just can't see or don't want to see that there is something wrong with what they're doing, and what they've always done. It makes sense, then, that you have to be careful as you approach meat eaters — you can't just stand up on the dining room table and lecture people about the horrors of the meat industry or call people "murderers" and dump fake blood on them, because you'll just end up alienating everyone and creating enemies because they won't understand your outrage. As a new vegan you may be extra angry or saddened by what you've just learned that made you go vegan, and you may be tempted to lash out at people who eat meat because it will feel cathartic. This reaction is entirely understandable in the face of so much horror, but there are much better ways to get people to realize what veganism is really about. The approaches we advocate won't earn you mad street cred with the PETA kids, but they'll do something more important: they'll help people to respect you in the long run, and as a result, they'll be more likely to take you and your crazy-ass animal rights ideas more seriously.

General Advice for Dealing with People

Given everything we just discussed above, you might be wondering right now if your choice to become vegan is worth all the hassle in dealing with not only figuring out what to eat and buy, but also figuring out how to deal with the people in your life. We're here to tell you that it's really not that bad, it gets much easier with time, and it's completely worth it. You're going to get a lot of stupid questions, but in among the stupidity you'll also find a lot of curious and well-meaning questions. You're going to get people who make jokes and make gross noises as they eat their meat in front of you, but you're also going to get people who go out of their way to make sure you are fed. You may even get someone to start thinking more about where their food comes from — and who knows, maybe they'll eventually go vegan! Although you can never predict how someone is going to respond, keeping some general advice in mind can help you get through most interactions you're likely to have with people. We'll go through some general advice first, and then we'll talk more about dealing with specific types of people, like family, friends, co-workers, vegetarians, and ex-vegans. A lot of this advice comes from years of experience in dealing with many different types of people, from books we read when we first went vegan, and from talking to other vegans and hearing stories of how they dealt with difficult situations. If we had to sum up our advice in a few words, it would probably come down to this: you need to be a happy, confident vegan who knows how to take care of yourself without being an asshole. But don't run off with just that! Let us explain more thoroughly.

DON'T BE AFRAID OF THE WORD VEGAN: As we said in Chapter 1, don't ever be afraid to call yourself a vegan. If people ask, tell them. As tempting as it can sometimes be when you walk into a restaurant where everyone is tucking into dead animals, you probably don't want to sit down at a restaurant table and shout "Hey everyone, I'm a vegan! Fuck all you murderous meat eaters!" because people will just look at you funny and think you're crazy. Instead, when people inevitably ask you about what you are eating and not eating, you can explain to them that yes, you are a vegan. Don't bother with trying to slide around the issue for whatever reason by calling yourself a vegetarian, a (god forbid) "veggie," or saying that you eat a "plant-based diet." If you are a vegan (and really a vegan, not a so-called "vegan" who eats cheese one in awhile), then be proud of that fact and secure in your choice to be a vegan. For your veganism to have the maximal impact in the culture you live in, people have to know you're a vegan. You defeat a significant part of the logical machinery of veganism as a protest if you're afraid to say that you're one of us.

BE KNOWLEDGEABLE IN YOUR VEGANISM: People are going to ask you why you are a vegan, and you should have an answer for them that makes sense to you. The answer will vary depending on who you are talking to and why, but you should probably have a few stock answers in mind so that you can respond to the question easily. For instance, you may just want to say "for animal rights reasons" or "for ethical reasons" if you want to keep it simple, or you may have a longer explanation in mind that goes more in depth for people who are really interested. People are also going to ask you tons of more detailed questions about being vegan, your health, and about animal rights arguments, and you should probably think about what you would say in those situations beforehand. There's lots of information in this book to help you, and you can check out one of the many references we mention throughout as well. People will know you are serious about veganism when you can answer their many questions, and that you are not just participating in a passing fad. This can be especially helpful when dealing with family, as we will discuss below.

BE PATIENT: As we discussed above, most people just don't get it. They don't see the world the way you see it. Be patient with them. Even though you'll most likely want to throttle people when they ask you the many deeply inane questions they seem fond of asking, take a deep breath, and answer the best you can. Remember that (chances are) you weren't always vegan, and you probably had tons of questions prior to being vegan that now seem silly to you.

DON'T ARGUE ABOUT VEGANISM OVER FOOD: While you may love to talk about factory farms and the horrors of milk and eggs, doing so while dining with meat eaters really isn't the time or the place to do so. You may get your jollies by watching meat eaters squirm when you point out the dead animal carcass on the table, but it doesn't always have the impact you hope it will. Fighting about veganism over food turns people off and makes them even more defensive about their choices. Instead of thinking like grown adults through the problems with what they're eating, most people just get angry with you. If people ask you questions, it's best to answer briefly or to talk in vague terms. Don't give up the discussion altogether, just put off the conversation for a more appropriate time. You can say something like "I'd be glad to talk about it more, but it would probably be better to do it after we eat." If the person seemed to be genuinely interested, there's nothing wrong with following up with them later.

DON'T BE A VEGANGELICAL: People really don't want to be lectured at or preached to. If you adopt the moral high ground when you talk to meat eaters, they'll quickly grow tired of you and shut you out. You'll just be seen as the condescending know-it-all fun-killer. Being preachy just creates anger and division, and puts people on the defensive. It can also often make people hostile towards veganism generally. In short, don't be a crass, annoying pain in the ass. The world doesn't need yet another one of those. We have plenty already, thanks.

LET OTHERS TAKE THE FIRST STEP: At least initially, let others come to you about veganism. Sometimes people have a genuine curiosity and would like to know more about what it is like to be a vegan, or they have a hard time understanding what being a vegan means. If people come to you with questions about veganism, answer them honestly and politely. This doesn't mean you can't be proactive about having a vegan potluck and inviting non-vegan friends, organizing a vegan group, or showing a film about vegan issues in your community, nor does it mean you should hide the fact that you are a vegan. It just means that you shouldn't be preachy.

NO BRUTE FORCE: This point is related to the previous two. Since most people don't get it and/or are genuinely curious, shoving your veganism down their throats isn't going to get people to respect you or to really understand what veganism is all about, since they'll most likely be turned off by your behavior. You can still be a proud, happy vegan who isn't afraid of calling yourself a vegan without forcing people to listen to your diatribes. This is especially true for family. Lecturing Aunt Edna on the suffering on egg farms while she is eating an omelet is just going to make her feel judged, alienated, and/or angry, and she'll most likely just tune you out and love that omelet even more. The times when brute force tactics are appropriate are few and far between, especially when you want to remain on good terms with the people in your life. Plus, people tend to value ideas more if they come to them on their own terms, especially at first. If you're too busy ramming leaflets down the throats of your friends and family, you're probably not the world-class activist you think you are. You might, however, be the joke everyone seems to be laughing about when you're not around.

DON'T GET UPSET WHEN TAUNTED OR TEASED: People can be mean, and people can be stupid, and more often than not, people can be both mean and stupid at the same time. Remember that because not eating animal products puts you into the category of freak, you suddenly become a target for those who like to pick on people for sport. Just wait until you hear someone tell you "oh yeah, I'm a member of PETA — People for the Eating of Tasty Animals." There are also plenty of assholes who will stare you in the face, stab a piece of meat with their fork, jam it into their mouth, and make sounds of utter pleasure as they eat dead flesh. (And of course they always think they're the first genius to have come up with this particular taunt. Are all bullies this stupid?) As we showed with the Uncle Bill example at the beginning of the chapter, you can't let these people get to you. The more you respond, the more power you give the person doing the taunting, and the more they're likely to continue. There are some really sick shits out there who, because they couldn't find any elderly people to push into traffic, get their jollies from this kind of annoying behavior. If you react, you're giving them their fix. For many of us, letting this kind of idiotic behavior go is difficult, but it is better for your mental health to just let it slide on by. Plus, remember our earlier point: if you react and get upset and angry, you're giving them what they want. Instead of feeding the moron, go to your own little happy place with this nice little mental exercise. In your mind, dress the bully in some ridiculous costume. A clown suit may do, or maybe if the particular bully fashions himself a "man's man," you could dress him in something he'd find incredibly emasculating, perhaps an extra frilly tutu. Put the tutu-clad bully inside a cage. And now, on the outside of the cage, hang a big sign that says "Please don't feed the asshole." Yes, this is a weapon of the weak, and it is probably nowhere near as cathartic as putting your vegan steel-toe boot into his smelly, omnivorous junk would be, but there's no need to waste your energy on these people. You need it for those who matter, those who will be receptive to the ideas. The fools are just in the way, and the sooner you begin to realize this, the sooner they become less and less relevant.

Along similar lines, if you get the reaction "ew, that looks disgusting" or "that's made of soy? Ew gross, I would never eat that" to your food, just shrug it off (unless they're your good friends who have a sense of humor, in which case you can come up with a witty retort right back to them about how disgusting their food is). People tend to look at our food as if it is toxic, as if somehow the lack of meat and dairy turns it into something that will jump off of the plate and attack them. Truth is, they don't know what they're missing. And of course it always befuddles us that people can think that mock meats and things made out of soy or wheat gluten are gross, but have no problem gnawing on the decaying leg muscle of a dead bird. (Have you ever seen someone's plate after eating a batch of wings or after attacking a whole chicken? It looks like a bird massacre.)

TAKE CARE OF YOURSELF — DON'T EXPECT TO BE TAKEN CARE OF: We first heard this bit of advice from Carol Adams, and are forever grateful. It may seem simple and basic, but it is extremely important. No matter what the situation — going to a friend's house for dinner, going to a restaurant, or going to a catered event — don't ever expect that you'll get fed. Most people don't know what vegan means, aren't used to cooking for vegans, and get flustered when expected to do so. Caterers often forget to provide a vegan option, even if it requested beforehand, or provide you with something that's barely edible. If going out with friends, you may end up at a restaurant with very little on the menu for you to eat. We'll discuss this more in Chapter 4, but taking care of yourself basically means checking ahead of time as to whether or not food will be available and requesting it if it's not, bringing your own food, eating ahead of time or afterwards, and asking lots of questions. If you're going somewhere, just expect that you may not be able to eat much or eat well, and have a backup plan.

MEEK VEGANS SUFFER: Since you can't expect that people will take care of you, you often must make your needs known and be extremely clear about it. This involves asking a lot of questions and explaining what you do and don't eat. In the vast majority of situations, you can't just say that you're vegan, you must tell them that you don't eat any animal products, including meat, fish, eggs, milk products, honey, and cheese (you often need to mention fish and cheese specifically because some people don't put them in the categories of meat and dairy for whatever reason.) You need to ask questions about menu items. If you're not completely upfront with people about what you want, then you're likely to suffer. You cannot be afraid to ask questions and make your needs known. This may seem torturous or uncomfortable, especially for the extremely shy, but you have to get used to it. If you had an allergy, you would have no hesitation in asking questions to make sure your food didn't have an offending ingredient. You are not being a pain in the ass, you're just making sure that you get what you want and that your needs are met.

FOOD WINS PEOPLE OVER: The way to people's hearts is indeed through their stomachs. Cook vegan meals for the people in your life and show them that vegan food is delicious. Remind people through food that we vegans eat more than sticks, twigs, apples, and random yard scrapings. Most people really do have a hard time understanding what it is that vegans eat, so show them! If you're not one for cooking or entertaining and you don't live in the middle of nowhere, you could always take your friends or family out to a nice vegan restaurant as well.

BE POSITIVE AND HAPPY: We'll talk more about this in Chapter 4, but it helps to have a positive attitude, both when you're talking about your veganism and when you're out dining. It never helps to play the martyr or to be absolutely miserable when the food situation may be less than optimal. Be a good example of a healthy, happy vegan, and you may get people to think twice before they criticize — and you just may also get people to realize that being vegan isn't impossible either.

Given the guidelines we've outlined here, let's look at how they play out with specific groups of people: family and spouses, friends, co-workers, vegetarians, and ex-vegans.[1]

Family (or, Am I Really Related to These People?)

Family can be the toughest thing about going vegan, and many vegans hesitate to announce their veganism to their family. Reactions range from support and outright acceptance, to neutral ambivalence, to more potentially difficult situations that include threats ("eat this or else..."), teasing ("mmm ... juicy steak"), and lengthy complaints and arguments ("you don't love my food so you don't love me"). Sadly, there's no single way to deal with these problems. Part of the issue is that every family is different, and despite what you might hear, there is no such thing as a "normal" family. You have to work in a way that's going to be the most effective in your situation.

At the outset, you should consider how food creates unexpected emotional attachments, and how food is also used to define roles. Bob's mom, for example, loves to cook for everyone. She loves having tons of people in the house, and she enjoys feeding them until they're on the verge of bursting. Knowing this, people do indeed come from all around the neighborhood to eat, because Bob's mom always has plenty around, and if she doesn't, she'll actually run out and get you something. This creates a welcoming environment and you get fed incredibly well — too well, perhaps! The problem is that by becoming vegan, Bob complicated this role for his mother. In his veganism, he made it more difficult for her to find fulfillment by preparing tons upon tons of food for him. What was once an enjoyable thing for her became an annoying challenge. "What can I make ya, hon?" became "Jesus Christ, you are so goddamn impossible to please!"

In all honesty, Bob's mom has been incredibly supportive of our veganism, but initially it all threw her off when it came to her expertise as a cook and as a provider. Because Bob's relationship with food changed, Bob's relationship with his mom was also changing in subtle ways. Over the years, Bob's mom has bought lots of vegan cookbooks and has gone online to look up recipes and new restaurants to try, and she always makes us an excellent meal every time we go over for dinner. Still, it took some time to get to this point, and you shouldn't be surprised if someone in your life sees your refusal of certain foods as an affront to their cooking or them personally. Remember that you might be challenging a long-standing role and that any change takes time and patience if

it is to be meaningful, particularly in parent-child relationships, regardless of age.

One thing that might help smooth things over is explaining to
your family that you are not going vegan just to reject them
and their family traditions. Sit them down and explain to
them that you are going vegan because you can't eat animals
any more, knowing what you know about the system of
animal agriculture — how in depth you go here is up to you,
depending on what your family will tolerate. You can still eat
mom's favorite pasta, just without the sausage. You can still
get enchiladas from your abuelita, just without the cheese.
You can still come to Thanksgiving dinner, you just won't be
eating the turkey or anything made with butter. In fact, the
best thing you can do is show your family that it is possible to
eat "normal" meals, just with vegan versions of everything.
You can also show them the possibilities and deliciousness
of other types of vegan meals in time, ones that showcase
vegetables rather than meat and dairy analogs (see Chapter
4 for suggestions).

Sitting down and explaining yourself may seem daunting and
make you feel vulnerable at first, because you are more likely
to be particularly sensitive to reactions about your decision
when you first become vegan. After time, you can roll your
eyes at the thousandth time you hear someone say, "no way I
would ever eat that shit," but at first these kinds of comments
hurt, and it's difficult not to overreact and get very upset.
Because family members are your family (regardless of
whether or not you are close to them), they often feel like they
can be extremely straightforward with you and tell you whatever is on their minds, even if it comes at the cost of insulting
you. You know that what you are doing is serious and has
purpose, but it may be difficult to explain this to your family
without getting overly upset at the static you may receive.

To counteract some of this, when you talk to your family, be confident and knowledgeable, but not preachy and lecturing or completely confrontational. You may be tempted to rage against your family and call them animal killers every time they eat meat, but this really doesn't help your situation. The occasional confrontation may happen (this is family, after all, and who doesn't have disagreements with their family?), but you may need to tone down the confrontation if you want to maintain good relationships with your kin. There's no better advertisement for your certainty about veganism than your being secure in your choice and communicating that to others. To this end, as we mentioned in the previous section, it helps to do as much research as possible before talking to your family, and to really understand the reasons why you are vegan so you can answer everyone's questions with solid answers. This also helps you counteract challenges from your family that come in the form of "concerns about your health." You'll hear the litany of perceived problems: "How will you get your calcium/protein/iron?" "Will you die if you don't eat meat?" "Can you just live on vegetables alone? It seems so unhealthy." "Aren't humans meant to eat meat?" Do some nutritional research not only to help fight these concerns, but also for your own good, so you can eat a well-rounded diet (more on this in Chapter 4).

Your goal should be to get your family to understand a little more where you are coming from, but don't expect that they'll change for you or ever completely understand why you are vegan. Most of them won't. They'll probably eventually be more accepting, but chances are they won't go vegan or really ever get it. At the very least, having done research will show your family that you are serious about your decision, that you know what you are doing, and that this is not just a passing fad, a typical reaction by many families. There are two ways to read this reaction:

A) THE GENEROUS READING

Perhaps readers of our generation went through a "phase" where they liked acid-washed jeans and Orchestral Manoeuvres in the Dark, or maybe they went through a "phase" where they wore parachute pants, beat-boxed, and saved their allowance for a square of linoleum for break dancing.[2] Or, maybe they went through a skate-punk phase that they never quite grew out of.[3] Whatever the case, these are legitimate fads. Like any other person, you probably got sucked into a few of them. But if you're vegan, and vegan for the right reasons, as we discussed in Chapter 1, you're likely not into veganism as a fad, but as a deeper expression of your ethical choices. This is why there's simply no reasonable comparison between acid-washed jeans and veganism. However, this doesn't mean this is how your family will see it. To them, your newfound veganism is likely as capricious as your love of those god-awful hideous parachute pants. They didn't get why you wanted a square of linoleum for break dancing, and they probably don't get why you'd give up what they see as tasty and delicious animal products. So when you tell them you're a vegan or that you're going vegan, they probably read you through their own lens of their own experience with you and your previous forays into territory they didn't necessarily "get."

B) THE UNGENEROUS READING

Your family assumes you're essentially incapable of making any long-standing decisions on your own; they view you as an immature child, and expect that your life is governed by fickle, ill-formed whims. Having made such silly choices from your heart and not with your logic, they expect that you'll eventually come around, see the light, and go back to your meat-eating, egg-sucking, milk-loving ways.

Far be it from us to tell you which one is more likely in your situation, but you should be aware of this potential reaction and how to respond to it. While it may seem like this is advice for teenagers,[4] it is true for people of any age who have to deal with parents or older adults in their family. To many omnivores, veganism looks like the worst kind of diet — a life without animal products just seems not worth living, as pathetic as that seems to us on the flip side. Coming from this angle, they'll view veganism as some kind of diet with near-religious strictures and wonder how anyone could keep at it for so long. The best way to deal with this is to be knowledgeable about veganism, and to stick to your beliefs.

If you ever do want people to take you seriously, you can't give in to coercion, pressure, or your desire to avoid conflict. Although you may think it is easier to just eat the lasagna that your grandmother made for you rather than try to explain to her why you don't want to eat it, you're doing more damage than good. You're sabotaging your own veganism to please others, and you're showing them that what you are doing doesn't really mean anything. Plus, once your family members realize that coercion works, they'll never stop (remember — meek vegans suffer). Although it may seem excruciating at first to say no to granny and it may seem like not such a big deal just to pick the cheese or meat out of that salad, standing your ground will provide more benefits in the long run. Eventually, people will get more used to what you do and don't eat, there won't be as many awkward moments, and they'll come to terms with the fact that you are serious about what you are doing.

To help ease the transition at first, offer to cook for yourself, whether it's for an everyday meal or a special occasion. You can't expect to be taken care of, especially at first, nor can you expect for people to just automatically start making you separate dishes. While it would be wonderful if your family catered to your every vegan need, many people just have no idea what to make for you now, and it doesn't even occur to most people to think about having vegan versions of margarine or milk around, or to not offer you the parmesan cheese to put on your pasta. For most people, it would be downright rude not to offer you something that they are offering everyone else, while for you it seems downright rude for people to be offering you meat or cheese when they know you're vegan. Most family members don't do this just to insult you, they just really have no idea what to do with you, and have a hard time adapting to your new needs. If it turns out that people do want to make you something, help them out by showing them where to find recipes you would like. Buy your own soymilk or coffee creamer to have around. Make your own food or cook for others without complaining about it. As we keep saying, all of this gets easier over time for everyone, you included.

Holidays can be especially difficult, because there are a lot of expectations and traditions to deal with, and everyone's nerves are on end anyway from all the stress of preparation and annoyance at having to listen to Uncle Pepe's stories about his hernia operation for the fiftieth time.[5] You may be lucky, and your family will offer to make you a tofurkey and your own bowl of mashed potatoes with soymilk and vegan margarine, but regardless, you should always offer to bring or make your own dishes to a holiday event. You can also ask if they'll make versions of various side dishes without butter or other dairy, but it's best if you make sure for yourself that you'll have something to eat. Don't expect people to change their holiday plans or to go out of their way to accommodate you. If you do get accommodated, make sure to be extra grateful. If you find that you just can't stand looking at the dead bird or pig or other offending section of animal that is the centerpiece of the celebration, either sit as far away as possible (maybe at the kiddie table), or if your family is extra gracious, ask them to cut the meat in the kitchen and just bring in the pieces to serve. You may, however, want to consider starting your own vegan traditions for holidays. While we love our families dearly, Thanksgiving is usually a bit too much for us, and instead of visiting either one of our parents' houses, we started hosting our own vegan Thanksgiving celebration, usually finding one or two other vegans to share it with. You could always do this, and then go visit family after the bird is eaten and the leftovers put away.

As you can see, the trick to dealing with family is being knowledgeable and being patient, and remembering that while it may be incredibly easy to get frustrated with their lack of understanding, their teasing, or their general irritation in response to your decision, it will take time for everyone to adjust. There are many factors with family and food that complicate the situation, but given time most families are likely to come around. After all, they're your family, and you're stuck with them and they're stuck with you, so you should try to make it work.

What Happens When Your Partner Isn't Vegan

We were lucky enough to have gone vegan at the same time, after we had already gotten married. Many people, however, find themselves in the sticky situation of making the choice to go vegan, but not having their partner and/or children follow in their footsteps. This can be extremely difficult, because more often than not we want our loved ones to have the same values we do about the things that matter most to us. When they don't share our vision of the world or don't understand where we are coming from, it can be disappointing and alienating.

What vegan wants to sit there and watch the people they love most stuff a dead animal into their mouths, knowing what we know about why it is so wrong? Not to mention, who wants to kiss someone who just chewed on a piece of meat?

Of course, the best solution would be to have your significant other go vegan, for the sake of your sanity and family harmony. As you might guess, however, this doesn't always happen, despite many arguments and attempts to convince them otherwise. Chances are, they'll get extremely defensive. Many partners see this change as threatening, too difficult, too much against the status quo, or just plain crazy. Others don't want to be seen as having been coerced by their partner — this is especially the case for men whose wives or girlfriends have gone vegan, because veganism is not seen as very "manly" in our society.[6] Another big problem is that many partners will feel like the person who has decided to go vegan has changed too much.

While many of these situations sound like they automatically spell disaster for a relationship, don't get discouraged. Lots of people out there make it work with a non-vegan partner, and we've learned a lot from talking to couples in this situation. The biggest piece of advice is to be patient with your partner, and ask that they be patient with you. You may want your partner to jump on the bandwagon right away, but if it's something they've never considered or thought about, then there's no reason why they should be immediately receptive to your arguments. Explain your reasons for going vegan without sounding accusatory. If they're open to learning more about why you decided to go vegan (and it may take them some time to get to this point), then give them suggestions of things to read or listen to that might help them understand your position. Pick materials that you know will suit them well — for example, don't give them graphic pictures if you know it will just turn them off and make them dig their heels in further. Sometimes hearing the information from someone other than you will actually make all the difference. In some cases, the partner will actually become vegan, but it may take time. In other cases, your partner will never be vegan, but will be supportive and understanding of your choice if she understands a little about why you are doing it, even if she can't make the choice for herself.

The second good piece of advice is to not coerce, nag or make deals with your partner to convince him to go vegan. If he is doing it just for you and doesn't really understand the moral and ethical reasons for doing so, chances are he will resent you and won't stay vegan in the long run. This is not a good situation to be in, obviously, even though it may sound good on the surface to have your partner be vegan. If it is going to work, you can't have a situation in which one partner feels like they are being forced to be something he or she is not.

Make sure you set ground rules in your house so everyone understands what you expect of them and what they can expect of you in terms of food and other household items. If you are the primary cook for your family, you need to find a way to explain to them why you are no longer going to be cooking or buying non-vegan things for them. You also must decide on how vegan the household will be. Will your family be able to eat non-vegan things in the house, as long as they prepare them themselves? Will they be able to bring non-vegan food into the house at all? If you're not the primary cook, then chances are you're either going to have to start cooking for yourself, or somehow convince your partner to cook you a vegan meal. Outside of the house, you will have little control over what the others do and do not eat and can't really force them to make vegan choices. Most likely, if you are all going out as a group, you will only be able to request that you all choose a restaurant that might have some options for you.

Setting up an atmosphere of mutual respect in this situation may seem impossible when your family thinks you're a crazy zealot and you think they're murderers, but with patience, time, and a lot of discussion, you can get there.

A Quick Note About Raising Your Children Vegan

We know many vegan couples who have raised completely healthy and happy vegan children from conception, and other couples in which at least one parent is vegan, who have made the decision together to raise their children vegan. They manage to deal with the complexities of birthday parties, school lunches and treats, day care, Halloween, and play dates with aplomb. Other people give their children the choice to become vegan, and some of the children do, and some of them don't. Still others insist that their children be vegan while they are in their house whether they like it or not. Whatever the situation, be aware of this fact: you will likely get an extreme amount of static about your choice not only from family members, but also from complete strangers. Many people think that you are going to do long-term damage to your child by raising them this way not only in terms of their health, but also in their socializing (because being vegan makes them so "different"). People can actually get quite nasty to you whether they know you or not (just ask brave parents who talk about raising vegan children on the web about the kind of comments they get[7]). So obviously, it is imperative that you are knowledgeable about nutrition and vegan diets if you decide to raise your children vegan not only for your child's well being, but also for your sanity in trying to counteract some of the wrath. The American Dietetic Association states that "raising a child vegetarian is healthful and beneficial so long as the diet is planned appropriately"[8] and it is quite obvious to anyone who has seen an energetic, smiling vegan kid (who is most likely ahead of the growth curve for his age) that this is the case. You should be well versed in the ADA's statement, since you are most likely going to have to mention it in response to concerns from your pediatrician, family, and others. You should also check out Dreena Burton's cookbooks and blog[9] — she has advice on what to feed children at all stages of life, and is raising three beautiful vegan children herself.

In addition to concerns about your children's diet, people will also accuse you of "brainwashing" your children, or "forcing your views on them." This is a ridiculous notion, and it is usually based on the fear that your "radical vegan views" are causing the young ones harm. Assuming that you are feeding your children well, this is a critique without merit. Parents are by definition people who should be passing their values on to their children. If you raise your kids to be feminist and non-racist, few people outside of the crazier pockets of Limbaugh-loving Republican America would accuse you of brainwashing them, or forcing your values on them. To the contrary, you'd probably be respected for your excellent parenting. If most people would not view your raising your kids as nonracist or nonsexist as your pushing your values on them, why is it somehow a problem to raise your kids as an antispeciesist?

To counteract some of the idiocy, it may help you to seek out a community of other vegan parents either in real life or online. There you can swap stories, find support, and give each other advice on how to deal with other people and difficult situations.

Why Am I Friends With These People Again?

Friends. Who needs 'em, anyway? Well, as it turns out, most of us do, and since they're the people you spend your free time with, you're going to have to deal with them. At some point, you're bound to end up in a situation that involves eating, and you're going to have to talk about your veganism. If you're lucky, you already have cool friends who are big-hearted, love you without question, and take your veganism into account when choosing a restaurant or preparing a meal. If you're unlucky, your friends just suck. By "just suck" we mean that they think you're insane. They may tease you, ask you stupid questions just to be annoying, try to slip meat into your food, and give you a hard time in general about being too difficult. Or, perhaps they will just look at you funny.

Regardless, you have to be prepared for the fact that your veganism can change the way that at least some of your friends relate to you. When we first told our friends that we had become vegan, some were supportive and wanted to find out how to cook us vegan meals, some were curious and asked a lot of questions, and others looked at us as if we had just told them that we were going to name our first child George W. Bush Torres. These friends could never fathom why in the world we would want to do such a thing, and in all the time that we knew them, they never ended up understanding it. Consequently, we ended up hanging out more with the supportive and curious friends than the disgusted friends, which was a lot easier for all of us. Additionally, because we were vegan, we also made other, new friends that we never would have gotten the opportunity to know in the past.

Although there are many similarities in how you can deal with friends and family, the old adage of you can choose your friends but you can't choose your family[10] makes the situation a little different. You pretty much have to figure out how to deal with your family, but when it comes down to it, you have more of a choice as to how to spend time with your friends, and you sometimes have a little more leeway in how straightforward you can be. If it turns out that they just can't handle a dinner with you as a vegan, then you either need to figure out other things to do with them, try to make it work out some other way, figure out what it is that is bothering them so much, or just count your losses and move on. And while it still holds true that you shouldn't be the vegan-gelical asshole to your friends, sometimes you can go a little further in explaining the whys of your veganism to your friends than you can with your family. If they're good friends, they'll listen and while they may not understand, they can often be supportive. But, you can't expect that the reactions of your friends to be all that different than the reactions of the rest of the world on this matter, even if your friends are among the most accepting people in other areas.

But, as we said above and we'll say again, meek vegans suffer, so you really do need to be up front with your friends about your veganism. If friends are throwing a dinner party, it is best you should explain exactly what this means in clear terms (e.g. "I don't eat meat, eggs, dairy, or fish.") It isn't that we think your friends are dumb, but you can't assume up front that everyone knows what veganism is. If you make this assumption, you might end up sitting in front of a dish covered in cheese. Offer to bring something with you, because then at least you have one thing to eat if all else fails. And if you think there won't be much for you to eat, just have a bite to eat ahead of time so that you aren't starving. When you offer to bring your own food, you remove the burden for the host if she was planning on cooking stuffed buffalo head or whatever the latest gourmet torture-filled dish of the week is, and you also have the opportunity to showcase a great vegan meal so you can demonstrate to others that veganism isn't just about eating yard scrapings. If you're lucky enough to have friends who are up to the "challenge," they'll make something special for you or change the whole menu to make you feel welcomed.

On the other hand, maybe your friends aren't so receptive. Maybe they're the kind that hit you with the million hypothetical situations ("would you eat meat if..."), chew steak loudly in your face, yell at you, hide meat or dairy in your food, or give you a really hard time about being too difficult. In this case, our advice is simple: tell them this is your choice, and you expect them to respect it. Give them some time to come around, but don't tolerate too much bullshit, particularly if they're hiding non-vegan things in your food. Be firm but polite, and don't let the teasing get to you. You should stand up for yourself, but don't get sucked into stupid arguments, especially while you're eating.

If you've been patient, polite, and non-harassing, and your friends still give you shit about being a vegan even after you've asked them to give you some leeway, you might need to find new friends. It's normal for people to be curious with a million questions or to be a little angry or defensive, but it's not right if they just can't let it go. It may sound harsh, but if you're into veganism for the long haul and you're serious about your ethics, you need to have friends who support your decision without giving you crap. The occasional bust or joke isn't anything to "dump" friends over, but if you're constantly being bombarded with stupid comments and the like, you need to make a stand, tell your friends how you feel, and tell them they need to stop. If they don't take you seriously, there's likely something wrong with your relationship, and apart from psychological issues that we aren't qualified to diagnose, there's no reason to stay in a relationship — friendly or otherwise — that is abusive. Veganism is a big part of any vegan's life, and those close to you should respect your decision.

This doesn't mean that you have to dump all your omni friends and get all vegan friends. As we know from experience, many of your friends will be accommodating and accepting. Plus, they will understand more what veganism is all about with you as a role model. But sometimes you just need to talk to someone who "gets it," to help you feel not so lonely and misunderstood. Depending on where you live, you may be able to find a local vegan group that does potlucks or meets up for dinner, or does other kinds of social activities — just search around on Google to see if you can find anything. If there's not one nearby, you can always try to start one up and see what happens! You never know, there may be some other fellow vegans in your area who are dying to meet other vegans. There's plenty of vegan camaraderie online as well, as we mentioned earlier in the chapter — join a forum, start a blog and read other blogs, participate in a chat, etc. Being able to really be yourself around other vegans can be refreshing after spending time out in that non-vegan world.

When it comes down to it, dealing with friends is pretty much like dealing with anyone else — you need to balance your forthrightness with some flexibility, and sometimes you have to take some shit you might otherwise not want to put up with. But when it does come down to it, most of your friends will likely come around to at least a passing acceptance of your veganism. Remember: it pays to be polite but firm, to stand up for yourself, and to avoid lecturing. With some luck and perseverance, you'll be able to get along just find with your non-vegan friends.

Does Someone Have a Case of the Mondays?

Workplaces provide you with a plethora of situations in which vegans get to be the freak: when you're at the annual company barbecue and you're standing around with your hands in your pockets because there's nothing to eat; when you're at a business dinner discretely trying to ask the waiter questions because there's nothing on the menu that looks vegan; when standing in line at the workplace cafeteria hoping the one vegan option isn't disgusting; when declining the invitation from your co-workers to go to a steakhouse; when not partaking in the communal birthday cake; or when sitting in your office eating the lunch you brought from home because the break room smells like ass after someone decided it would be a bright idea to microwave their fish leftovers from last night. However it shakes out, there's almost never an end to the suckfest.

These vegan freak moments can go in many different directions, depending on who you're with. Soon after becoming vegan, Jenna had to attend an annual get-together with her co-workers. Luckily, she was able to speak to the person organizing it and order a special vegan meal beforehand (no way was she about to spend the obligatory $25 for the meal and not be able to eat any of it!). But, at the event, everyone else's meal was already set out on the table, and Jenna's meal arrived separately and late, since the kitchen nearly forgot about it. Of course, everyone at the table soon noticed that one of these things was not like the other, and the questions commenced. "So, you're a vegan?" Just as this question came, another person asked what a vegan was. Jenna patiently explained that she doesn't eat any meat, dairy, or eggs. "So, where do you get your protein? Your calcium? You're young now, but it's never too early to think about osteoporosis." Given this, Jenna really wanted to launch into a discussion about how vegan diets are actually better at preventing osteoporosis because they have plenty of calcium, and too much animal protein can leach calcium out of your bones, but she bit her tongue and gave the standard answer "it's no problem to get protein and calcium" and mumbled something about beans, tofu, and leafy greens. "So are you vegan for political reasons or some other reason?" Jenna responded briefly, saying "for animal rights reasons primarily, health secondarily." Then for some reason the discussion turned to the South Beach diet and how yummy free-range meat is, although apparently bison is a little bland. One person even made the comment "I guess happy animals taste better." Jenna desperately wanted to shout "they'd be a lot fucking happier if you didn't eat them!" but since the focus was off her, she instead carried on a conversation about gardening and herbs with the person sitting next to her.

On another occasion, Jenna was at an important business dinner at a restaurant that was vegetarian-friendly, but had nothing on the menu that was vegan. She didn't want the clients to think she was a total freak, so she was nervous about drawing too much attention when ordering. She asked the waitress if one of the dishes on the menu was made with any eggs or dairy, and she said, oh, you're vegan? I'll check with the chefs. She came back, and said that the dish did indeed have eggs and dairy in it, but they could make a special dish with white beans and kale. Great! Only the person sitting next to her noticed she didn't order something off the menu, and simply said "oh, if I had known you were vegan, we could have gone someplace more vegan-friendly!" Jenna responded by saying, "oh, really, it's no trouble! I have plenty to eat." Later during the meal, one person at the table went around to see what everyone else had ordered and asked how they liked their dish. They got to Jenna, and noticed that it was something not on the menu. They figured out that it was vegan, but their reaction was more of "oh, so, is the dish good?" and that was it! No twenty questions, no weird looks, no drama.

Although we are proud to be vegans and would gladly have a discussion with anyone interested, the workplace is just one of those realms where you really have to learn to pick your battles, or you'll end up going crazy and ostracizing yourself from others, and lose a chance to show others how great being a vegan can be. As we've already stated, being confrontational may have its time and place, but work is rarely that place. Once you reveal yourself as a vegan at work, you're going to get a lot of different reactions. Some people will be incredibly accommodating, even overly so, and will try to make sure you are well taken care of. (One of Jenna's bosses once even printed out a list of vegan-friendly restaurants in the area of a conference so she would have something to eat!) Others will ask you the same familiar stupid questions that will drive you nuts and try your patience every time. Some will tag you as a freak and make fun of you or even try to get you to eat meat, just like family and friends. Others will insist on talking to you about hunting, fishing, and the great barbecue they went to last weekend where they ate a pigeon stuffed into a duck stuffed into a chicken stuffed into a turkey. A lot of what goes on depends on the kind of work you do and the setting in which you work. You may be in a place where you never interact with your co-workers around food, and it may not really be much of an issue. Or, you may have to deal with cafeterias, communal lunch areas, or going out to eat with clients or co-workers on a regular basis.

As with family and friends, with co-workers it's important to remember the guidelines outlined above. Discussions about veganism at work will most likely come up over food, so being confrontational while eating will just make people defensive. You will most likely be asked many questions over time, some curious, some stupid. By being patient and not letting the stupid comments get to you, you may actually get people thinking, or at least understanding a little more about what veganism is all about. Be solid and happy in your commitment to being vegan. You never know, maybe for your birthday they'll actually get you a vegan cake. Or, they'll be dicks and order you a non-vegan cake that everyone can eat except you.

But your birthday's not about you, silly. It's about cake. Duh.

One place you don't want to get into a discussion about veganism is over a business or client dinner (unless your business directly has to do with veganism). If it comes up in this situation, the best strategy is to just cut the conversation short, politely, of course. You're really not going to get any converts in this type of environment, so just go for being a good example of a happy vegan. Ask the questions you need to ask in order to be served a vegan meal, but don't make a big scene or be confrontational. If you don't get served a great meal (or much of a meal at all), don't act all pissy, either — just deal with it and get something to eat afterwards (see Chapter 4 for more advice in this realm).

If you find that you have to eat at an event for work, try to find out ahead of time where it will be and call the caterer or restaurant and see if they can accommodate you, or talk to the person in charge of the event and see if they can order you a special meal. If you are going out for a casual meal with co-workers, try to suggest that everyone go to a place that you know has at least one option for you, rather than to a steakhouse where you have to smell all the dead flesh and eat nothing but a baked potato without butter. Bob has used this strategy with success to go to a Chinese buffet rather than a deli with his former colleagues. If you're somewhere where you don't have much to choose from, eat what you can and then grab something afterwards. If you haven't already discussed your veganism with your co-workers, answer any questions that come up politely, even though some of them might be so irritating that you want to bang your head repeatedly on the table. Again, don't make it look like you are suffering to be vegan, even though you know it's annoying as hell to be in a restaurant that doesn't cater to vegans.

On a day-to-day basis, it's probably easiest if you bring your own food with you to work (including lunch and snacks), since you'll know you have something to eat, and you'll know it's vegan. If you're organized, you can make a large batch of rice, pasta, soup, sandwich filling, or salad-type dish on the weekend and take portions of it for lunch during the week. We know this sounds soccer-mom-like, but trust us, it is worth it, especially if you want to eat healthy and not be starving by dinner time every day, or if you want to avoid spending lots of money at a restaurant. Planning ahead also avoids the "shit, I overslept and have no time to make lunch before work" situation where you end up either making peanut butter and jelly for the thousandth time or hoping you can buy something nearby. Bring little containers of applesauce, pretzels, chips, fruit, carrots, hummus, nuts, granola bars, or whatever else floats your boat for snacks so you don't have to rely on the vending machine (remember, you can't read the ingredients on anything in a vending machine before you buy it), cafeteria, or local restaurants or stores. All of this will probably save you money in the long run, too, since it is cheaper than eating out. You can even get yourself a cutesy retro lunchbox or a fancy Japanese bento box system if you're into that sort of thing.

Jenna found one unique plus to taking her own lunches to work every day — people started asking questions and being interested in what she brought. As soon as she was done heating her lunch in the microwave, the secretary would say "oh, that smells good! What is it?" and even sometimes ask for the recipe. If people understand what it is that vegans do actually eat (see Chapter 4), they can start to grasp that we're not all malnourished freaks. This, of course, can also backfire on you, and get people to tell you how disgusting your food looks even when it is not even remotely so. You may hear something like "how can you eat that shit?" as they are stuffing their mouths with dead animal muscle or miscellaneous animal parts. (And yet we're the weird ones. Go figure.)

If you're in a situation where you have a workplace cafeteria (and this goes for university cafeterias as well) and there aren't many (or any) vegan items, you can often talk to the administrators in charge and ask that they carry at least one vegan item on their menu every day. They may ignore you or make something kind of gross, or they may come up with great meals. It's always hard to tell how it will turn out, but it's worth a shot.

AS WE SAW WITH FAMILY, FRIENDS, AND CO-WORKERS, being vegan around non-vegans can be a test of your diplomatic prowess, not to mention your patience. But trust us, we have found from experience that being non-confrontational with people you have to deal with on a regular basis can actually open their eyes — even if just a little — to veganism. While many interactions can be annoying, it's important to remember that it's not all bad; we've had wonderfully accommodating friends, family, and co-workers that have provided us with great vegan meals or made sure we had something to eat, even though we insisted that they didn't have to worry about us. As time goes on, people may become more receptive and even go out of their way to learn more about veganism, to figure out how to cook vegan meals, and maybe even buy their own vegan cookbook or two.

Dealing with Vegetarians and Ex-Vegans

It may surprise you that the most shit you will receive about being vegan will most likely come from some vegetarians and ex-vegans. Then again, if you already know some vegetarians and ex-vegans, this may not shock you at all. Even though they seem (at least on the surface) to hold kindly views towards veganism, many vegetarians have a hard time bridging the gap between the differences between veganism and vegetarianism, and many ex-vegans seem to hold a grudge. This of course is not true of all vegetarians and ex-vegans — we've met some who have been extremely supportive, friendly, and cool about our veganism. But there are a minority of ovo-lacto vegetarians who will enjoy harassing you or will view you with suspicion and doubt. They'll scan you for leather (even though they may be wearing it), quiz you on the extent of your veganism, and look for any cracks they can find in the foundation of your veganism. They may call you a radical or dismiss you for going "too far" with your vegetarianism. After all, in their minds, why would you be a vegan when milk and eggs don't directly kill animals (and they taste 'oh-so-good')?

In some ways, this kind of reaction isn't all that much different than what hostile meat eaters sometimes do to attack us, and that's not a coincidence. In both cases, the ultimate goal is to be able to dismiss us and our choices through a constant dissection. If they can break us down in even one place and show us not to be the pinnacle of compassionate perfection that they expect, then they can dismiss us, at least in their own heads. Somehow, if they can trip us up, they can call us hypocrites, and return to eating their Eggs Benedict.

Another part of what's going on here is feeling that we're being judgmental. Granted, some vegetarians do have run-ins with judgmental vegans who annoyed the hell out of them; but even if you aren't being preachy, you can still be perceived as someone who thinks that they're better than everyone else, only because you're doing something different than vegetarians. In essence, your choice to avoid what they're eating is perceived as judging them. When vegetarians meet you and learn that you're vegan, they're forced to remember why it is that they're vegetarians, and they have to ultimately confront why they're not vegans too. In that instant, your very presence has likely forced them into some tough thinking. All at once, they've got to come to terms with why they're not vegans, decide if it's something they want to think about and deal with, and then also decide how to react to you. If they're really into their cheese/milk/eggs/etc., then the initial reaction may be something like "wow, I'm a vegetarian but I could never be a vegan. I just don't think I could ever live without my cheese/milk/eggs/etc." This in an understandable reaction, particularly if the person doesn't know many vegans or understand the ethics behind veganism.

Other ovo-lacto vegetarians may want to paint you as the freak (yet again). As we mentioned before, if they can conveniently but you into a category of "radical" or "freak" in their brains, then they can adequately dismiss you, and subsequently dismiss your choices too. Ovo-lacto vegetarians have actually asked us, "don't you think you're taking this just a bit too far?" This is their way of sticking you into a little box that they can deal with and conveniently ignore. Against our expectations, this kind of reaction is more intense in 'mixed' company of omnivores and vegetarians, when the vegetarian doesn't want to be seen as marginal, radical, and far-out as you. It is the way the vegetarian communicates to the rest of the group, "hey, I'm okay, I'm not nearly as weird as the vegan!"

So how does one respond to these kinds of problems? There's a lot to be said for standing up from the table, giving everyone the finger, and flipping the table over as you run out of the room calling everyone "murderers" and proclaiming the need for animal liberation.

Or perhaps not.

Seriously, the best way we've found to deal with this is just to let it go. That goes against our ethos most of the time, which is generally to say what's on our minds regardless of the consequences, but in this case, it won't help (just like we describe above in our encounters with family, friends, and co-workers). One of the best responses we've found is a simple "this is my choice and it might not be right for you, but I feel better this way. If you're curious, I'd be happy to talk to you about it." Surprisingly, something that simple can be incredibly effective and even disarming.

It bears mention here that if you're already a vegan, you should be kind to vegetarians regardless of what you think of their choices. We're not saying you should collapse if confronted on the question of animal cruelty and how it relates to eggs and milk, but we are saying you should maybe think twice before getting frustrated. One characteristic common to all vegans is that we're passionate about what we're doing. We're the "converted" in a sense. We take our choice to be the sensible one, and some of us get frustrated when we see others not doing what we know is right. We've seen this shirt on the 'internets' that has the word "vegetarian" with the "etari" cut out (resulting in the word vegan) and the slogan underneath says something like "Cut out the crap. Go vegan." We think this sums up how many vegans feel, but we can't forget that the vast majority of vegans were vegetarians first. If we do forget and get pissed at vegetarians for not coming around quickly enough, we run the risk of being judgmental idiots who scare people off of the good thing that veganism is.

In our case, we've found ourselves annoyed beyond words with vegetarians who've sat in a room with us after a lecture decrying the horrors of the dairy industry that they continue to support through their consumption of — get this — milk products! Grr. We wanted to stand up, give them the middle finger, flip the table over ... oh wait, sorry ... ummm, we actually wanted to stand up on our chairs and scream at them, "HOW CAN YOU KNOW THIS AND STILL DRINK MILK, YOU COMPLETE IDIOT?" but decided against it. (Can you tell that we like the idea of standing up on stuff to make a point?) Had we done this, we'd be nothing better than the unpleasant judgmental vegan, we'd be asking them to make choices on our terms rather than their own, and we'd probably be fucking up their possible movement towards veganism on their own terms (which is the only way to go, we think). We're not going to lie: we would love it if everyone were vegan. But yelling at people, calling them on their contradictions, and challenging them isn't always the best way to approach the issue. For one, it personalizes things in ways that aren't always helpful and makes people feel attacked and marginalized. For another, it makes you look like a complete bastard with nothing better to do and it lets people dismiss both you and veganism.

Like mom used to say, patience is a virtue. Rather than lecture vegetarians, be a good example of a vegan, and continue to educate them about animal exploitation and oppression when appropriate. We let people come to us on our terms, and then from there, we work with them as their interest dictates. Again, it sometimes goes against our very real desire to scream sense into people, but we've found this to be more effective. This less confrontational strategy works because there are a number of thoughtful vegetarians who will never stop thinking about veganism after they've come to discover that it is possible, with you as an example. For others, they may never get beyond where they're at, but in this world of limited time and resources, your energies are best spent on those who have the best chance of becoming vegan rather than badgering the hell out of someone who will likely never make the step. In either case, it can't hurt to cook for them if you're halfway decent at it.

Before we call it quits for this section, there's yet one more kind of vegetarian annoyance to deal with: the unrepentant ex-vegetarian or ex-vegan. We're not talking about folks who were once vegetarian and now want to return to vegetarianism; if nothing else, these people are usually your friends. No, we're talking about a different kind of creature, a different kind of beast born of weakened and misplaced commitment. We're talking about the loudmouthed ex-vegan.

The unrepentant ex-vegan is usually one of those people who went vegan for the wrong reasons (most of which we listed in Chapter 1), but seems to think that there's something inherently wrong with veganism, not themselves, that made it so untenable. Unfortunately, they have a penchant for being extremely vocal about their displeasure, and many of them seem to have unfettered access to publishing their viewpoints in newspaper columns for some reason. These people who "just couldn't live without sashimi" or who "felt horribly sick" or who just couldn't hack the peer pressure may seem like just another annoyance out there, but the problem is that they make veganism seem difficult or impossible, and make vegans out to be deprived, miserable fools. As we know from experience, veganism is neither difficult nor does it make us feel deprived or miserable; but to many omnivores who don't know any vegans, these stories make it appear that way. In fact, many omnivores want to believe that it is impossible and horrible, because then they have an excuse to not think about it. As vegans, we want to show people there is life after meat, dairy, and eggs (and a good life at that), and people do not have to suffer to live by their principles. Ex-vegans sabotage that message at every turn, because they allow people to dismiss vegans by making us look intolerant and misguided. The lesson here is twofold: first, make sure that you're going vegan for the right reasons and take care of yourself once you do, and second, if you do have a run in with an ex-vegan in person, the best remedy is to show them a great example of a happy, healthy vegan who has no regrets.

Embracing Being Vegan and Freaky

As we said in Chapter 1, it is important that you embrace both the vegan label, and the fact that you are a freak in a society where eating animals is the norm. This stance may make you feel lonely sometimes — you feel like you're the only one in the world who cares — especially if you live in a remote area where there aren't a lot of other vegans around, if any. In addition to this, some new vegans get extremely saddened by the horrors that they've just learned about, and can't stop thinking about them. These two things together lead some people to just want to sit around at home and sulk and revel in their misery. This doesn't do anyone any good, especially the animals that you're so concerned about. You need to remember that it is a non-vegan world and prepare yourself to deal with that fact. You also need to remember, though, that every new vegan brings us one step closer to a more vegan world. You can't ever hope to bring about that world if you're sitting at home playing the martyr. If you find yourself getting into a funk, remember that there are other people out there like you. Refresh yourself by hanging out virtually with other vegans online — join a forum, find a chat room, join a group on Facebook, start a blog and read other vegans' blogs, or just search around for vegan websites.

Facing the challenges of a non-vegan world may seem overwhelming at first, but once you get the hang of how to deal with other people, you can feel confident in your choice, and show the world that veganism is possible, easy, and the right thing to do. We can't always please everyone, no matter how hard we try. As you go through the various trials and tribulations you'll face as a vegan freak, you must remember the reasons that you've chosen veganism, why they matter, and why you need to stick with veganism despite the crap you'll get. Though you may be painted as an extremist radical who wants to challenge all that is right and good in the world, you must remember that this is but a defense mechanism on the part of your accusers. As long as omnivores can continue to consume without knowing or thinking about the conditions of exploitation involved in production, they can fool themselves into thinking their conscience is free and clear. Through your veganism, you remind them that this transaction isn't so simple, and most omnivores want nothing less than to have to think about where their food comes from.

When people give you a hard time, remember that you're living by your conscience, and that is never simple. On our blog, Bob once wrote the following entry about dealing with omnivores:

> ... some [omnivores] see fit to call me an extremist. Me? I'm just living by my conscience. If I'm to be true to my ethics, this is what I must do. Yes, it meant giving up blue cheese (which I loved, though which now seems gross), ice cream (though Soy Delicious rocks my socks), and cream in my coffee (soymilk works just fine, thanks) but these were the only choices to make since I couldn't in any way justify daily consumption of products that caused so very much suffering. Once I made myself think about it (which took some time, admittedly), there was no other way to go.

Bob knew, and couldn't un-know.

Regardless of how people view you, regardless of the personal problems that veganism might create, you must remember that you too know, and once you do, it becomes impossible to un-know.

This is something you cannot change for anyone.

Notes to Chapter 3

1   It may sound like we occasionally repeat ourselves in this chapter, but we wanted to apply the above information to different situations, and we wanted cater to the people who may want to skip a section or just go back and read a particular section for reference.

2   For the record, neither one of us went through either of these phases. Honest. Do you think we'd ever admit to them so publicly if we did?

3   This phase, however, Bob owns up to.

4   If you are a teenager, you may want to check out the book *Generation V* by Claire Askew. A teenager herself, Claire gives plenty of advice for dealing with parents while still living under their roof, as well as navigating other typical teenage vegan minefields.

5   In truth, Bob never tires of hearing Uncle Pep's stories about his hernia operations. He could, however, do without having to see the actual bump itself.

6   What real men eat tofu, anyway, right? Real compassionate men, that's who.

7   For a great example of the views of a vegan parent raising a vegan child as well as other vegan-related news and reviews, check out Vegblog.org.

8   http://www.vegetariannutrition.net/articles/Vegan-Diets-For-Children.php

9   Dreena goes into detail about feeding children in her book *Vive le Vegan*, but also check out *The Everyday Vegan* and *Eat, Drink, and Be Vegan*. Dreena's blog is at http://vivelevegan.blogspot.com.

10 Or is it that you can pick your friends, and you can pick your nose, but you can't pick your friends' nose? Or you can if you're really gross?

CHAPTER 4

WHAT DO VEGANS EAT ANYWAY?

AT SOME POINT OR ANOTHER in your time as a vegan, you'll end up hearing the inevitable "SOOOO, what do vegans eat anyway?" question. The best you can hope for is not to hear it so often that you want to throw a block of extra-firm tofu at someone's head. Even so, it actually is a fair question, one which you may even be wondering yourself if you're new to veganism. With no meat, fish, dairy, eggs, honey, or animal by-products, people often wonder: what's left to eat? Our usual answer is — everything else! There are so many negative stereotypes out there about what a vegan diet is like: it tastes like cardboard; it's nothing but plain, unseasoned tofu and salad; it's like rabbit food; it's grass, twigs, and other lawn clippings — and therefore (because we only eat yard rubbish) vegans are all pale, skinny, malnourished, and deeply unhappy people. Many people we talk to think we must have will-power of steel to be able to eat the way we do, and we often hear comments like "I could never be vegan — it's too hard" or "I like steak or cheese [or insert some other product of death here] too much." Frankly, we don't find a vegan diet hard to follow at all, and we certainly don't have any super-powers or anything. One thing we do have, however, is a healthy and positive attitude towards the way we've chosen to live our lives. Yes, that sounds a bit new-agey (peace, man!), but it is undeniably true that if you have a positive outlook on what you're doing, and you fully understand the reasons for it, being vegan is liberating and empowering. The rest of the world sees our diet as deprivation, but we see abundance. They see it as limiting, we think of it as liberating. They see it as annoying, we see it as necessary.

This attitude can go a long way in showing non-vegans our point of view — that you don't have to suffer to live by your ethics — and make you a much happier, confident vegan in the process. In this chapter, we'll discuss this attitude some more, as well as how to get yourself cooking great vegan meals in no time, how eating vegan can be extremely healthy if you're careful about what you're putting in your body, how you can navigate your way around the grocery store without going crazy, and how to survive restaurants and traveling without starving.

Abundance, Not Deprivation

Okay, be honest with us: how many times in the last week have you eaten a peanut butter and jelly sandwich? If this is your go-to sandwich for lunch (and maybe even breakfast and dinner as well), then you need to expand your vegan horizons a bit! When you first become vegan, it is easy to rely on the foods that you already know and love that happen to be vegan, but you may be at a loss as to how to go beyond PB&J, french fries, or pasta with marinara sauce. You may also be throwing your hands up in despair as you are listing off all the things you can't eat now that you've made the decision to go vegan.

Our first piece of advice is to stop thinking about it as what you can't eat: think of it instead as what you will and will not eat. We just don't want to eat meat, dairy, and eggs — to us

CHAPTER 4: WHAT <u>DO</u> VEGANS EAT ANYWAY?

it's not a matter of can't. We obviously could eat animal products if we wanted to — there's nothing about vegan anatomy
that makes this impossible — but we choose not to because
they don't fit in with our ethics. When you think about it like
this, you're not depriving yourself of anything. Instead, you
are making a choice that comports with your stance on the
world. Suddenly, meat, dairy, and eggs are not really even
in the category of food anymore. Thus, you're still eating
whatever you want — you just don't want to eat anything that
came from an animal.[1]

This focus on the possible and the positive — on living your
ethics and making decisions based on your values — not only
puts you in the right frame of mind to approach veganism, it
also orients you to an entirely new and wonderful world of
what you can and want to eat. With most of us living in
societies that focus many meals around animal products of
some kind or another, it is too easy to forget how much else
is out there, but really, the variety is yours for the taking as a
vegan, contrary to what might seem like common sense. To
understand this, think about what the average omnivore
eats — one day chicken, next day something from a cow, next
day something from a pig. Typically, there's a side of some
sort of starch, and if you're lucky, a vegetable makes its way
in there too — there's really not much variety at all. But picture
the wide variety of vegetables and fruits that are in the
typical produce section, even in a small grocery store. There
is an array of colors, tastes, textures, and smells that you can
open yourself up to — there are hundreds or thousands of
new vegetables to try. We've found that over the past several
years, we've eaten a much wider variety of foods than we
ever did as omnivores or vegetarians, and we've come to
learn a lot more about herbs, spices, and seasonings as well.

So What's for Dinner?

Cooking might seem to take on a new challenge when you are a vegan, but it also takes on new meaning. You're preparing meals that reflect your ethics, that prove that you don't need animal products to eat well (or for that matter, to be healthy), and that can highlight the abundance of foods available to vegans. If you haven't done so already, one of the first things you should do is get yourself a copy of a good vegan cookbook. If you can't buy one for whatever reason, borrow one from a library or a friend, or look online at a site like vegweb.com that has a ton of free recipes to choose from, or at one of the many vegan food blogs. Try to find a cookbook that suits the way you like to cook and eat (i.e. do you like comfort food? International flavors? Quick and easy meals?). Having one or many vegan cookbooks can help you in several ways: they can teach you about ingredients you might not have heard of before (and even tell you where you might be able to find them), they can help you visualize new meals that don't contain animal products,[2] and they can help you to not eat the same thing day after day. You can exist as a vegan on hummus, potato chips, and soda, but you can't do it for long without feeling like crap and potentially damaging your health. Armed with your new cookbooks, you'll be inspired to try new dishes and new foods, and see all what veganism has to offer.

Buying a cookbook might seem like common sense to many, but as we've learned, there are a lot of people out there who just don't like to cook or who don't know how to cook. Our advice to these people is that if you really want to stay vegan and if you want to be healthy, now is the time to get over your fears or hang-ups and learn. You'll undoubtedly thank yourself later. Despite what Oprah and her chefs might make people think, vegan meals don't have to be time consuming, expensive, ingredient intensive, or complex. In fact, often the simplest preparations are the tastiest — for example, we often stir fry a large bunch of cabbage or broccoli as a side dish, with salt as the only seasoning. You'd be surprised at how good it is. Of course, if you want to learn to be a vegan gourmet chef you can do that too, but it's not a requirement for everyday vegan eating. You may need to enlist the help of a friend or family member, a few cookbooks, and a lot of trial and error, but the more you cook, the better and faster you'll get at it.

You might also be scared off by one of the stereotypes of vegan cooking that has hung around over the years: it is bland and boring. Unfortunately, people who either don't know much about vegan cooking (i.e. most omni restaurant chefs who think that vegans only eat oily pasta with roasted vegetables) or who choose to follow the 70s hippy paradigm[3] of vegan cooking (i.e. plain grains and beans and no spices) continue to perpetuate this stereotype. Although meals not loaded with cheese or meat may taste different to you at first, it certainly doesn't mean that what you are eating is inferior or is doomed to be tasteless and boring. The more you cook vegan meals, the more you'll come to appreciate and under-stand the beauty and taste of vegetables and how they can be paired with herbs, spices, and other seasonings to liven your palate.

But what do you do if you don't like vegetables? Some of you reading this may be shaking your head at this question, thinking, "how can anyone who doesn't like vegetables become a vegan?" Despite every common sense notion to the contrary, we know there are a bunch of vegan vegephobics out there, because a lot of them have sent us email over the years. If you count yourself among those who develop a severe case of the howling fantods at the thought of eating lots of vegetables, there is hope. Chances are that your affliction stems from some relatively simple issues, like your having grown up not eating a lot of vegetables, having a texture issue with them, or having had them prepared horribly. Whatever the cause, we urge you to give peas a chance. (Ha! Give peas a chance. Get it?! Okay, look, we're bored, and in our late 30s, and we're writing a book for fun. We have to amuse ourselves some way or another, so you get cheap puns.) In all seriousness, make an honest effort to try some vegetables again, this time in earnest, and with an open mind. As you age (and the longer you're vegan), your tastes change, and things that might have seemed unpalatable in the past may suddenly taste good to you. Jenna used to hate raw cucumbers and tomatoes, but now she eats them with abandon. You should also try them prepared a different way than you've had them in the past. If you've hated mushy, cooked carrots, try them raw. Try lightly steamed and seasoned or stir-fried broccoli rather than broccoli cooked to death or raw. If all else fails, you can try to "hide" foods in smoothies or in pasta sauce so you can be sure you're getting some of the nutrients you need without having to see or taste the offending food.

Whether you love or hate vegetables, in looking through your new cookbooks, think about new ways of conceptualizing a meal. Rather than just substituting a meat analog for dead meat on your meat-starch-veg plate, look into one-dish meals, new ways of using beans, legumes, and grains, and new ways of mixing vegetables. Investigating various types of international cuisines can definitely help: for Mexican food, you can throw together a bunch of vegetables and beans and throw it all in a tortilla for a tasty and filling burrito; for Indian food, you can make a legume dish and a veggie dish and eat them both over rice or with flatbread; for Chinese food, you can stir fry a ton of vegetables and tofu or seitan and eat it over rice or noodles; for a Middle Eastern meal, you can have falafel, hummus, couscous and vegetables, and any number of salads. You can even reinvent a typical Western meal, changing the focus from meat to what were formerly the side dishes. And don't forget that you can always make a main dish out of a soup, salad, or sandwich if you make them big enough and throw on a ton of ingredients that you like.

Of course, you can still go the 'fake meat' route as well. Veggie burgers come in many flavors and textures, and are readily available in most mainstream grocery stores. You can also get substitutes for ground beef, sausage, turkey, chicken strips, patties, and nuggets, ribs, and bacon. If you are lucky enough to find an Asian grocery that has specialty fake-meat products, you will also be able to find mock seafood. Many of these products are soy or wheat based, so they aren't great for people with those allergies, but you may be able to find veggie burgers that are based on rice, vegetables, and nuts instead (and you can always make your own!). You should also experiment with tofu, tempeh, TVP (soy textured vegetable protein), and seitan (wheat gluten) as substitutes for meat in dishes like stir-fries, soups, stews, and chiles, just to name a few. Luckily, many of these items are available in well-stocked grocery stores as well as health food stores and co-ops, or you can find them online.

Non-dairy cheeses have come a long way in the last few years, and are becoming more readily available all the time. In the past, you could only find some pathetic, slimy, off-tasting cheese substitutes that you had to put with cooked foods to be able to stomach, but now there are some that are so good that you can eat them as a snack with crackers. They've even reached the Holy Grail of vegan cheeses — ones that can melt and are great on pizza. If you can't find any of these vegan cheeses locally, (see the warning below about casein) you can order them online, or make your own fresh "cheeses" using ingredients like cashews, chickpeas, and nutritional yeast. You can also find vegan versions of just about every other dairy product you can think of, including whipped cream. One caveat that we should note, however; if you've recently become vegan, we suggest that you don't try any of the cheese substitutes until you've been vegan for a few months. They will inevitably taste "off" to you because they don't taste exactly like "real" cheese. To those of us who have been vegan for some time, however, they are the bee's knees. Wait — is it vegan to say bee's knees? Okay, they are The Shit. That's better. Regardless, speaking generally, it's useful not to think of "fake" meats and dairy products as a complete substitute for the dead animal versions you're used to — they have merit on their own, and are often good for getting that form-factor you might be in the mood for.

So if you're jonesing for a grilled cheese sandwich for lunch, there are options. Overall, speaking of lunch, sandwiches, soup, and salads are all brilliant options. You don't have to go for the meat or cheese substitute for a sandwich, but it can make life easy, especially at first. You can find vegan "lunch-meat" slices in most grocery stores these days (which vary from eerily meat-like to kind of meh), or try a sandwich or pita with hummus and vegetables, avocado and vegetables, a veggie burger, or a tempeh "bacon," lettuce, and tomato on toast. Make up a big salad with the works, and try some smoked or flavored tofu on top. Try some bean, grain, or pasta salads too. Or, make up a batch of soup at some point during the week and take some each day for lunch. Also, don't forget that you can always double a recipe for dinner and eat left-overs for lunch. And though it may mean some advanced preparation on your part, you may want to consider taking your lunch to work or school every day. Unless you're lucky enough to have a vegan-friendly cafeteria where you work or have a number of vegan-friendly restaurants nearby, you're going to be shit out of luck when it comes to finding something interesting for lunch on a daily basis. Plus, if you take lunch you'll be less likely to snack on that one kind of vegan potato chips in the vending machine.

But what about the most important meal of the day? Luckily, you can replace a lot of breakfast items with their vegan equivalents: soy, rice, almond, hemp, oat, etc. milk[4] instead of cow's milk on cereal or in smoothies, soy creamer for your coffee, veggie patties or bacon instead of dead pig, tofu scramble instead of scrambled eggs, vegan granola (with a vegan sweetener) and soy yogurt, a bagel with vegan cream cheese, vegan margarine, or peanut butter, vegan muffins and other baked goods, pancakes, waffles, or french toast instead of ones made with dairy or eggs, or you could eat fresh fruit, toast with nut butter or vegan margarine, oatmeal or some other grain porridge — or leftover vegan pizza! You didn't think that you could still eat all this stuff and have it be vegan, did you? Also, many cookbooks have excellent recipes if you're looking to try out new things that might seem daunting to veganize, like pancakes, waffles, French toast, or egg-based dishes like frittatas or scrambles.

Another thing that on the surface seems difficult to veganize are baked goods and desserts, because they so often rely on dairy and eggs. This, as many vegan waistlines know, is not the case — it is easy and tasty to veganize your baking. There are multiple cookbooks out there that are dedicated solely to desserts and baking, and plenty of delicious recipes in other general cookbooks. It's easy to substitute for the dairy — just use a vegan milk, vegan margarine (such as Earth Balance in the US), etc. in its place — but the egg gets more challenging because it acts as a binding and rising agent and gives many baked goods their structure and texture. You'll see that common egg substitutes include a product called ENER-G which is a powder that you mix with water, as well as soy yogurt, banana, tofu, or increased amounts of baking powder and baking soda included in the recipe. The "egg substitutes" that you can find in the dairy or freezer section of your grocery store are actually eggs (usually with the yolk/cholesterol removed), so you don't want to be using those. And fear not, chocolate addicts. You can still eat chocolate, just not cow's milk chocolate. Look for dark chocolate bars (not all are vegan — check the ingredients for milk), vegan chocolate chips at your local health food store or online (the ones in the regular grocery have milk), or chocolates with rice or soy milk.

Taking the time to teach yourself how to cook healthy vegan meals and figuring out what and how you like to eat is well worth the effort. It is cheaper and much healthier than eating out all the time, or than relying on pre-packaged, processed foods, unless you like being that stereotypical pasty vegan.

Being a Healthy Vegan or "Oh My God If You Don't Eat Animal Protein You Will Die a Horrible and Ugly Death"

"So where do you get your protein?" If you haven't heard that question yet, trust us, you will soon, and many, many times over. For some reason which probably has something to do with the meat industry's propaganda, people think that animal products are the only possible source of protein in the human diet. Oh yeah, and the only way to get calcium is to drink milk, and the only way to get iron is to eat red meat. And we need to eat fish to get omega-3s. When you talk to people about what you do and don't eat, suddenly everyone is a nutritional expert. They know — with absolute certainty — what is and is not good for you, and the thousands of ways you can die if you don't eat animal products. You'll hear about someone's cousin's friend who was a vegan and woke up one day to find that he was blind, or that he couldn't get it up, or that his fingers had fallen off, or that he'd turned into a giant insect in his sleep or something. However you shake it, there are a lot of nutritional fallacies out there about vegan diets, thanks in part to scare-mongering stories such as the claims that soy will make you gay,[5] delusional, or impotent, or that vegan diets kill children,[6] but if you sit down and thoroughly go through the research, you'll find that there's plenty of evidence that not only can a vegan diet be healthy, it can be healthier than the standard American (Western) diet if you do it right.

We are not nutritionists or doctors, nor do we play either of those things on TV. So to know exactly what your body needs to be healthy, we recommend that you run out right now to your favorite bookstore or local library, log onto amazon.com, or go wherever fine books are sold, and get a copy of *Becoming Vegan* by Brenda Davis and Vesanto Melina, who *are* professional nutritionists and registered dieticians. Go do it now! It's okay, we'll wait. Have your copy yet? Good. Read through it and keep it around for reference. *Becoming Vegan* is the go-to guide for vegans to know what nutrients we should be getting to stay healthy, and how to get them.

According to Davis and Melina, it is quite easy to live vibrantly and healthfully as a vegan if you keep in mind one important recommendation: eat a varied diet that contains enough calories to sustain you. You may find yourself falling into the trap of eating the same foods all the time (or existing completely on vegan junk food), but it is easier to get all your protein, vitamins, and other nutrients if you eat a wide variety of fruits, vegetables, grains, and legumes.

While you should talk to a professional nutritionist who understands veganism and/or read through all of *Becoming Vegan* to get a full portrait of a healthy vegan diet, we thought we'd highlight some important nutrients that you should make sure you're getting:

B12: This is the one vitamin that is nearly impossible to get in a vegan diet without supplements or fortified foods. In and of itself it is vegan, because it is produced by bacteria. The problem is that these bacteria are mostly found in animal guts (and thus the vitamin is present in animal products), and sometimes in soil, depending on how the soil is treated. You would think that since vegetables grow in soil they'd be able to pick up some of this B12, but it's not the case — despite what the freegans say, you can't rely on dirt as a vitamin source. Even if you eat foods fortified with B12 (like soymilk and nutritional yeast, for example), you should take a supplement at least once a week if not more, because you don't absorb all the B12 you ingest and you want to make sure you're getting your recommended daily allowance (RDA). Some vegans think they can get away with not taking a B12 supplement or fortified foods, but they are wrong. Among other things, vitamin B12 is essential for making sure our circulatory and nervous systems work correctly, and you wouldn't be of much use to yourself or to anyone else if those systems failed. However you look at it, vitamin B12 deficiency is serious, and preventing it is simple and inexpensive: just take a supplement that contains B12. You can even get small patches that are a little bigger than a 10-cent coin in the US which you can stick behind your ear or on other parts of your body (no, not there, you perv!). You leave them on for 24 hours, and you get your dose of B12 for the week. In any case, if you're concerned you're not getting enough or absorbing enough B12, ask your doctor to check your levels with a blood test, and consult with your doctor or nutritionist on how to best meet your B12 needs.

OMEGA-3s: You've probably heard that you should make sure you get them, but from where and why? There are plenty of plant-based sources of these fatty acids, which are essential for healthy cells and organs, and especially for healthy brain and nervous system function: flax seeds and oil, walnuts, algae, seaweed, hempseed, chia seeds, canola, soy, and some dark leafy greens. If you don't think you've gotten enough of these Omega-3 sources in your diets, try a supplement. To be completely healthy, you should look for a supplement that has sources of EPA/DHA fatty acids (which are mostly derived from algae or seaweed). Luckily, there's no need to kill fish to get this essential nutrient.

VITAMIN D: Recent research has shown that this nutrient may be more important for overall health than we thought (mostly by helping the body use the calcium it ingests properly). Humans can produce it in our skin with exposure to sunlight, but there are a lot of factors that can complicate how much we get (skin type, amount of exposure to sun, quality of sunlight depending on time of year, etc.). Besides sunlight, vegans tend to get most of their Vitamin D through fortified foods such as soymilk. If you're not drinking some sort of fortified non-dairy beverage, consider a supplement. One note: Vitamin D2 is vegan, while Vitamin D3 is animal-derived.

TRACE MINERALS: While it is easy to get most trace minerals in a vegan diet, if you avoid certain foods like nuts and seeds, sea vegetables, or certain other vegetables, or if you eat mostly processed foods, you may be lacking in important minerals like iodine, selenium, zinc, and even calcium. Either find ways of including a source of these minerals in your diet, or take a supplement that contains them. Contrary to popular belief, it is actually quite easy to get iron in a vegan diet, provided that you eat a wide variety of vegetables, legumes, and grains.

The more you know about how to get proper vegan nutrition, the healthier you'll be, and the more likely you'll stay vegan. You may have heard stories about some ex-vegan who thinks that veganism is pure evil because they got sick or felt horrible while they were vegan — when chances are they were probably not eating enough, or not eating the right things. Ex-vegan stories get a lot of press, unfortunately, because they uphold one of the myths about veganism that people really want to believe — that it's unhealthy and untenable in the long run.

The biggest and best piece of advice that we can give you is to not eat a junk food diet. Yes, that's right, we said it — put down the cupcake! Many vegans like to think that just because something is vegan, that means it must be healthy — after all, it doesn't have cholesterol or as much saturated fat! But by relying on baked goods and junk food, not only are you risking being deficient in some important nutrients, but you are also risking higher cholesterol, diabetes, and other diet-related diseases by eating a diet full of processed bad carbs, sugars, and fat. This doesn't mean that you need to be monk-like in your adherence to a whole-foods diet, but it does mean that you should try to include as many whole grains, legumes, and fresh fruits and vegetables as possible while not relying solely on baked goods, processed foods, or pre-prepared foods.

You're probably grumbling something right now about how we are killjoys or health food nazis because we tell people not to eat cupcakes every day and what the hell is wrong with deep fried tofu anyway? Well, we've learned from experience that what you put in your body on a daily basis matters. Save the cupcakes and the deep fried tofu for special occasions (and no, it just being Tuesday is not a special occasion) or once in awhile (and no, every Tuesday is not once in awhile). We like vegan junk food as much as anyone, but it's never a good idea to have it as a major food group in your diet, and we want you to be happy, healthy vegans.

For the record, when we say bad carbs, we mean refined flours, added sugars, white rice, and starchy potatoes. Good carbs are the cornerstone of any healthy diet — don't worry, we're definitely not going all Atkins on you here. Good carbs include whole grains, vegetables, legumes, and fruit. When you eat something filled with white flour and sugar, you're not only filling your body with nutrient-void, insulin-spiking food, you are also *not* eating something that is filled with healthy vitamins, nutrients, and fiber. Dr. Joel Fuhrman explains that when you eat nutrient-deficient foods, your body craves the nutrients it is missing, causing you to eat more.[7] Eating foods rich in fiber, antioxidants, and micronutrients will help you regulate your hunger better because you'll feel full when you are supposed to. In addition, these foods help you fight off diseases and illness by supporting your immune system, and help prevent chronic diseases associated with the Standard American Diet (SAD) such as heart disease, cancer, and diabetes. Plus, as you'll inevitably find out, eating a fiber-rich diet will make you more regular than you could ever think possible. Whether you want to or not, if you spend any time around vegans at all, you'll also discover just how much other vegans love talking about poo and their poo prowess.

So you don't think that we're just talking out our collective editorial ass here (nice segue, don't you think?), there's lots of research to back up what we're saying. For instance, Dr. Neal Barnard, who promotes the health benefits of a vegan diet as well as reasons not to experiment on animals, summarizes these types of studies on the effects of diet on health in his book *Dr. Neal Barnard's Program for Reversing Diabetes*. Although it is geared to people who are diabetic or pre-diabetic, the evidence Barnard cites and has collected suggests that following the advice in his book will also help you prevent high cholesterol, high blood pressure, and heart disease. If you didn't think that vegans could have all of those diseases, think again. A diet full of refined flours, sugars, and bad fats (like those found in processed foods) can increase your cholesterol and limit your body's ability to regulate blood sugar levels. By not eating antioxidants, micronutrients, and fiber, you also set yourself up for an increased risk for cancer.

In their book *The China Study*, T. Colin Campbell and Thomas M. Campbell really send home the message that a healthy vegan diet can prevent cancer. The China Study is the cumulation of many years of research of the effects of diet on health, which connected how people in various parts of China ate with the kinds of diseases they got over time. In the areas where the diet consisted mostly of whole grains, vegetables, and fruits, there were very few incidents of the typical Western diseases — diabetes, heart disease, cancer, etc. In the more industrialized or urban areas that adopted a more meat- and dairy-heavy diet that didn't contain as many vegetables and the like, there were much higher rates of these diseases.

So why do we care about you eating healthy anyway? After all, we're vegan for animal rights reasons. For one, the healthier you are, the more likely you are to be a happy vegan and to stay a happy vegan. And if you're going to be vegan, why not take advantage of the health benefits? Why not avoid the health risks of the SAD since you're not eating meat, dairy, and eggs anyway? A vegan diet loaded with vegetables, fruits, whole grains, legumes, and nuts, done right, is one of the healthiest diets on the planet. Eating healthy means that you'll have tons of energy, you'll feel more alert and happy, and you'll fight off illness better. If you do it right and add regular exercise, chances are you'll live longer too.

One of the most important things to remember with all of this is that you're not on a diet; you're changing the way you're eating. While people like Oprah and her fellow cleanse devotees can tell you that a vegan diet may help you shed a few pounds, doing it for that reason alone can get you in heaps of trouble and will likely prevent you from staying vegan in the long run. Remember to take care of yourself so you can be the happy, healthy, glowing vegan that you deserve to be. If you're ever unsure about whether or not your diet is healthy enough or if you're getting all the nutrients you should, consult a nutritionist or a doctor, and for the sake of all that is good and sensible, don't ask random (or even non-random) idiots on the Internet for advice about things as important as your health.

Surviving the Grocery Store

Surviving the grocery store is really a matter of learning how to read labels and knowing where to look for the products that you want. In fact, you can often spot a fellow vegan in the store — they're the ones standing in the aisle scrutinizing the ingredient list with a scrunched brow. But in order to help you become expert label readers, we'll need to clarify a few things about what is and is not vegan.

It's obvious from what you've read in this book so far that vegans don't eat meat, fish (it's not a vegetable!), dairy products, and eggs. But what about honey? And what exactly are the animal by-products to watch out for? Here's the definitive answer on honey: it's NOT VEGAN (add reverb here).[8] While some claim it's not a big deal, honey is an animal product, plain and simple. Bees are in the animal kingdom,[9] we don't need honey to live, and it's easily avoidable, so it's a no-brainer. But if you need more convincing ("but bees aren't harmed and they naturally make honey, right?"), think of it as this — honey is a product that bees make for themselves, and we are taking it away from them for our own use. This is much like how cow's milk is taken away from a calf to be consumed by humans, when you think about it. And, bees are inevitably harmed in the whole process. So why cause harm when you don't need to? Agave nectar is an excellent substitute for honey, and is completely vegan.

While we're on the topic of sweeteners, let's talk about sugar. In general, the white sugar you find in regular grocery stores is processed with bone char (yes, that's charcoal made from animal bones). Although there are no animal products in the final package of sugar, they are a vital part of processing, and therefore most vegans will not buy bone-char refined sugar for use in their home. There are plenty of alternatives to this sugar, however: beet sugar (which is white, but not refined in the same way as cane sugar), natural cane sugar (which usually has a slight brown tinge to it), turbinado sugar, and other types of sweeteners such as agave nectar, brown rice syrup, maple syrup, stevia, and molasses. High fructose corn syrup (and golden syrup), corn syrup, fructose, maltodextrin, and other sweeteners you might find in highly processed foods are also usually vegan (although they really are horrible for you!). Artificial sweeteners are just chemical concoctions and are vegan, although they have been extensively tested on animals.

Ok, back to label reading. You might be thinking, why do I need a lesson in label reading, if I just need to look out for eggs, milk, and meat? Because, unfortunately, there are many derivatives of animal products in food that aren't immediately obvious from their names. You can actually buy guides to animal-derived ingredients (such as *Animal Ingredients A to Z*) in book or pamphlet form or get free ones online or for your iPod that you can carry with you. If you live in Europe, Australia, or New Zealand, you can simply look up the list of E numbers to find out what the additives are in your food, and then research their sources. The list of animal ingredients is a long one, so we thought we'd just highlight some of the most common ones here.

Casein, whey, and lactose[10] are all derived from cow's milk. Casein and whey powder are milk proteins, while lactose is a milk sugar. You'll find all of them in various types of processed foods, especially breads and other baked goods, as well as snacks. Casein is particularly annoying, because many manufacturers put it in "vegetarian" soy or rice cheeses to make them melt, rendering them completely useless to vegans. Some products that contain casein, like coffee creamers, are even labeled non-dairy, which just blows our minds. It just seems so wrong that you can label something non-dairy if it has a dairy ingredient in it! So lesson is, if you are going to by a non-dairy cheese, please check the label carefully. The other thing to watch out for is whey in margarine. Most margarines you find in your average grocery store are not vegan because of milk by-products, so read the labels carefully, or look for Earth Balance brand in the US.

Gelatin is another very common animal product that is found in candies, Jell-O, marshmallows, and other processed foods, as well as gel-cap-style medicines and supplements. Gelatin is particularly disgusting, because it is made from the hooves and connective tissue of animals (blergh). If you are craving some of these usually gelatin-laden products (like Jell-O, gummy bears, or marshmallows) and cannot find any vegan versions locally, you can find plenty of them online at places like Cosmo's Vegan Shoppe. We'll discuss medicines in the next chapter, but you can also find supplements that are made with non-gelatin capsules online or in health food stores.

VITAMIN D3: As we mentioned above, vitamin D3 is animal-derived, while D2 is plant-based. You'll find D3 in many fortified foods like cereals; the problem is that sometimes it's only listed as Vitamin D in the ingredients, not specifying which kind. If you're not sure, write or call the manufacturer and ask.

NATURAL FLAVORS: These could really be anything, because the manufacturers aren't required to tell you on the package. Some companies will specify that their flavors are plant-based (especially if they are a company that typically caters to vegans), but most of the time you have to once again call the manufacturer to be sure.

It might sound onerous to have to be so vigilant when buying groceries, but at least you'll know what kinds of things you are putting in your mouth. The longer you are vegan, the easier it gets to read labels and find the brands that you know are vegan. But a good rule of thumb is that if you've never bought a particular item before, be sure to check the ingredient list carefully first, even if you've bought foods from same brand in the past. Another way to go is to not eat so much processed food in the first place. If an ingredient list takes up half the package and sounds more like a chemistry lab than food (or for you Europeans, has more E numbers than anything else), the wise thing to do is probably not eat it, even if it is vegan. By sticking to produce, whole grains, beans, legumes, nuts, and the like, you won't go blind from reading labels and you'll mostly likely be eating much healthier. But, chances are that you are going to want to buy some packaged food at some point, and knowing how to scan that label can save you a lot of time. Luckily, in the US anyway, manufacturers are starting to put lists of common allergens at the end of the ingredient list in bold (although not consistently), which often include egg and dairy. Check that bold list first if it's there; if it does say contains egg or dairy ingredients, you can put the package down right away, and if not, you can then scan the rest of the list for other possible animal-derived ingredients like gelatin, honey, and the like. But a warning — just because the bold list doesn't include the words egg or dairy in it doesn't mean that the product is vegan. Read the rest of the ingredients to see for sure.

Ok, now to the really important stuff that I'm sure you've been on the edge of your seat wondering about. What about booze? Or maybe it hadn't even occurred to you that booze might not be vegan because what the hell could be not vegan about fermented plants? Beyond the obvious like Irish creme liquor, many alcoholic beverages (especially beer and wine) are fined (filtered and clarified) using things like isinglass (the swim bladders of fish), albumen (egg), gelatin, bone char, or contain non-vegan ingredients like cochineal (crushed up bugs, yes, seriously), pepsin (pork), casein, lactose, and more.

There is some good news, though, in that there are vegan fining agents, and it isn't hard to find vegan beer. All German beers are vegan — there's a German Beer Purity law that has been in place since 1516 that dictates what can and cannot be in beer — and many of the major North American brands are vegan as well, including anything from Anheuser-Busch, Miller, Pabst Blue Ribbon, Rolling Rock, Sierra Nevada, Moosehead, Anchor Steam, and for those of you in the northeast US, Yuengling. So if you want to party it up with your PBR, you're good to go. It gets trickier with microbrews, British and other European beers (besides German beers), as well as Mexican and Asian beers, because their veganness varies tremendously. And — brace yourself, beer drinkers — Guinness found in the US is not vegan, although they tell us that in Ireland it is. Also watch out for honey in beer (it's usually obvious from the name of the beer).

Many hard liquors are vegan, though some have the fining agent problem or are colored red with cochineal. Wine can be a real pain in the ass because there are so many manufacturers and so many non-vegan fining agents and ingredients that can creep in there. Many of the organic wines are vegan, but not all.

If you are interested in finding out whether your favorite tipple is vegan or not, do a Google search for the many lists of vegan booze that other industrious vegans have compiled — there are a bunch, so there's no real point in listing individual ones here. Or, as with any other food you aren't sure about, call or email the manufacturer and ask if there's any animal-derived ingredients used in processing.

THE GOOD NEWS IS THAT IT'S EASY TO BE VEGAN anywhere in the developed world if you have access to a grocery store with produce, grains, and legumes. You don't need any fancy ingredients to be vegan, not even tofu. Certainly there are places that are easier than others to be vegan, but that is why the gods invented the Internets (or wait, was it Al Gore?). If you're willing to pay the shipping costs, you can have just about anything delivered right to your door, including fresh organic vegetables, vegan haggis (no offense, Scotland, but seriously, what the fuck?), vegan blue cheese, a 10 pound pail of nutritional yeast, and frozen faux shrimp. There are even several all-vegan stores that do all the label reading for you, such as Cosmo's Vegan Shoppe, Pangea, and Vegan Essentials in the US, as well as Viva Granola in Canada, the Cruelty Free Shop in Australia, and the Vegan Store in the UK, among many others; Google around and you'll find even more places to shop at that have what you need.

Eating Out

No, not that kind of eating out. Get your mind out of the gutter! We mean eating in restaurants. Ahem.

Going out to eat is one thing that is bound to give any vegan high blood pressure. We've heard a ton of gripes from our fellow vegans about their dining experiences: there's nothing on the menu to eat, there are no vegetarian or vegan restaurants near where I live, my friends /family/ co-workers are real assholes when we try to pick a restaurant, the waitstaff looked at me like I was diseased, they put cheese on my salad even after I said no cheese, they didn't think bacon was an animal product, I ended up eating a limp iceberg lettuce salad with a sad, hard chunk of greenish-pink tomato. Unless you're lucky enough to live in an urban area and only have all-vegan friends and family who only go out to all-vegan restaurants, you're bound to have one of these experiences yourself.

While dining experiences can certainly be frustrating, there are a few things you can keep in mind when going out to eat to help keep yourself sane, especially if you're going out with a bunch of non-vegan people. First, keep a realistic attitude and expectations. Second, remember that meek vegans suffer, as we discussed in Chapter 3. Third, as we said in Chapter 1, there is no Paris exception. And finally, be prepared and take care of yourself if you have to.

As Jenna can attest to (and Bob as well, who is usually on the receiving end of the pre-meal low blood sugar grumpiness), keeping a positive attitude in the face of hunger isn't always easy. But it is important to keep at least a realistic attitude towards your restaurant experiences. In general, we tend to expect the worst but hope for the best. Sometimes, you'll go out and your waiter or waitress will know what vegan means, and will take very good care of you. Other times, you'll find someone who doesn't realize that Parmesan is in fact cheese or who refuses to take back your food even when they screwed up and put some sort of animal product in it.

Expecting the worst but hoping for the best sometimes leads to surprising results. One weekend Jenna's grandmother and great aunt were in town visiting, and we needed to find somewhere to take them to dinner that would both suit their palates and give us at least something small to eat. In the rural wasteland we were living in, there were plenty of places we could have gone that would have made them happy, but with absolutely zero on the menu for us. We ended up choosing an Italian restaurant that we hadn't tried yet, hoping they could accommodate us. We were skeptical. At first glance, there was nothing on the menu that was vegan except maybe a salad. So, we started asking questions. We said to the waitress "Okay, we need to make what might seem like a weird request to you. We're vegan, so we don't eat any cheese or eggs or meat or any other animal products. Can you make us the roasted vegetable pizza without cheese?" Sure. "Does the crust or sauce have any dairy or meat?" Usually the sauce has meat, but we can substitute the vegetable marinara for the sauce. Huzzah! And you know what? It was a pretty good pizza, too. But the most amazing part? The waitress didn't look at us like we each had a third eye. She was incredibly patient, accommodating, and kind. As a result of the reasonable and kind treatment we received, we went back to that restaurant for our cheeseless pizza numerous times, taking other vegan and non-vegan friends with us, even though there was pretty much only two things at the restaurant that we vegan lunatics could eat. We always thanked the waitstaff profusely because they were always so nice to us, and we especially made sure to tip well so they remembered that being nice to us had its rewards. To put it most simply, we acted with civility, asked nicely, thanked graciously, and rewarded the accommodation appropriately. It worked out great for everyone involved: the waitstaff, the restaurant, and us.

This unfortunately doesn't happen all the time, but it does illustrate that you can be pleasantly surprised sometimes, especially if you're willing to ask a few questions, if you have the right attitude going into the situation, and you're extra nice to the waitstaff and/or kitchen staff. When you are making demands of waitstaff and kitchen workers, your requests can go a long way if you have just a little bit of sympathy with their situation. In general, in a busy restaurant, the staff is like an army that's waging a campaign to get out the most food in the least amount of time. Recognize that you may be interrupting this flow with your special requests, and try to put yourself in their shoes — they're just people trying to do a job. You never, ever have to apologize for what you are asking for, but being patient and treating people like human beings who are trying to earn a living rather than mere servants who should be commanded to obey your every wish will get you far in our experience. To put it in simple terms, solidarity and empathy counts for a lot. It won't always help, and sometimes, people can be real assholes regardless, but for obvious reasons it never hurts to be nice to the people who have control over your food (ever see the French toast scene in *Road Trip*? 'nuf said.) Regardless, you should probably just accept the fact that you're not going to have a perfect meal every single time you go out, but that's the case even if you could eat everything on the menu. If you do end up with just the salad or a plate of french fries, it doesn't help to sit there with your head in your hands looking miserable, complaining constantly. Shrug it off, enjoy the company you're with, and get something to eat afterwards.

Remember when we said that meek vegans suffer? It is especially true in restaurants if you're too afraid to ask questions. Okay, say that for whatever reason you find yourself in a restaurant where there's not a whole lot for you to eat, or there's something on the menu that looks like it might be vegan, but you're not sure. The only way to increase your chances of eating well that night (or, eating anything at all, really) and to decrease the chances of being served something non-vegan is to ask questions. You can't be afraid of inconveniencing people, looking weird in front of your friends, bothering the waitstaff, standing out, or whatever hangup you might have about the situation. If people think you're being a pain just because you want to know what you're about to put in your mouth, then they're the weird ones. The more you do it, the more you'll get used to it, and the more you'll know what to ask about. Meat and dairy are hidden in some surprising places (we've been to an Italian restaurant where they put butter in the tomato sauce, for example — have they never heard of olive oil?), and often it won't occur to restaurant staff that yes, things like beef stock, butter, and mayonnaise are actually animal products. If you see something on the menu that appears to be vegan, ask the waitstaff if there is meat, fish, milk, cheese, butter, or eggs in the dish (sometimes, you'll need to be specific — in the sauce? In the dough? etc.)? If a dish looks like it could be easily veganized, ask if you can get the dish without the lone animal ingredient or two that it appears to contain, after explaining to the server what you will and will not eat. Often they'll have to go back to the kitchen and check. If there's nothing on the menu that appears to be vegan and/or not easily veganizable, then ask the waitstaff if they can check with the chef to make you something that's not on the menu. This sometimes can turn out amazingly well if you get a chef that's up for creating something different, or it may be the kind of bland, boring meal that is apparently what some chefs think vegans eat all the time.

Putting your ethics aside so as not to appear a pain in the ass, or because you don't want to waste the food that someone accidentally brought you that has cheese in it, or because you don't feel like just eating the salad is not an option. If you're only vegan when you feel like it or when it's the most convenient (i.e. only at home), then why call yourself a vegan? There is no Paris Exception that makes any logical or moral sense. At the end of the day, you want your veganism to mean something, and it means very little if you sabotage it by calling yourself a vegan and then doing some very non-vegan things like eating cheese. Once you get used to it, being vegan in restaurants isn't hard at all and figuring out how to get yourself fed becomes second nature.

Yes, it's frustrating that you have to do some extra preparation, bug the waitstaff, and put up with bad food and annoying people, all while omnis get to go pretty much wherever they want and order anything off the menu, and don't have to go through much as much hassle to get a decent meal. But you can't let it get you too angry or frustrated. Remember, it's just one meal. You're not going to wither away and die if you don't get the best food you've ever had whenever you go out to eat.

Of course you'd love for every meal to be an opportunity to show your fellow diners what a great abundance of food vegans can eat, but unfortunately that just doesn't happen. But being the miserable vegan or the vegan martyr ("oh, sigh, I must eat like this for the animals") at the table doesn't help people with their image of vegans either. They'll go back and say, "see how miserable Jane was at dinner, and she didn't have anything to eat? I don't want to be like that. Being vegan seems hard. Look at everything she's had to sacrifice to live by her ideals." Instead, if you don't seem overly bothered by your paltry salad and fries or by having to ask a bunch of questions and if you seem confident in your choices, you won't perpetuate the miserable vegan stereotype and you won't trigger as much of that kind of reaction from your fellow diners. Remember, it's just one meal. If you do want to convince your family and friends that vegans can and do eat well, invite them over to your house and cook them up something good, bring an awesome dish to the next potluck or get-together, or take them out to a restaurant that you know has great vegan food.

The best way to make sure you aren't going to be miserable despite your best intentions not to be is to make sure you take care of your own needs. This might mean having a snack before dinner (yes, we all know what mom used to say about not ruining your appetite) to stave off hunger pangs in case there's not a lot for you to eat at a restaurant. Or, it might mean planning on having something to eat after dinner somewhere else or at home, just in case. It might mean calling ahead to the restaurant or catering company (for special events) to ask if they have anything vegan or if they can make you something special. And when traveling, it often means bringing your own food (see the next section for more details). Hell, even if you aren't traveling, sometimes bringing your own food or supplies can help. Having a Larabar stashed in Jenna's purse has saved us on numerous occasions from having loudly growling stomachs. We even know of other vegans who bring their own condiments, bags of vegetables, beans, etc. in a manbag or purse so they can make an extra big meal out of some rice, potatoes, or salad that they can get at a restaurant. It sounds like a lot to do (one of the advantages of going out to eat, after all, is not having to prepare your own food), but if you know you're going to someplace like a steakhouse with your family and can't get out of it, then having a semi self-catered meal will help you from starving and being miserable — and you've taken care of yourself.

Another way to take care of yourself if you're in a group trying to pick a restaurant for the evening is to try to convince the people you're with to go to a place that has at least one or two things on the menu that you might be able to eat. It doesn't have to be a vegetarian or vegan restaurant (although it's great if you can convince your fellow diners to go there), just somewhere with options. In urban areas, it's not hard to find places with veggie burgers (but ask about dairy and eggs in the burger and bun) or some sort of veggie sandwich or pasta on the menu, and you have a wide range of international restaurants to choose from. In rural areas it might be a little more challenging, but you'll get a lot of chances to practice your new question-asking skills.

Looking for international restaurants might give you more options for things to eat than steakhouses or restaurants with typical American (or Australian or British) fare, but be aware of a few things that are not vegan in places you don't expect:

- **CHINESE:** Chinese restaurants almost always have at least a small vegetable section on their menu, and probably even have a tofu dish or two. You don't have to worry about dairy too much here, but ask about meat stock in the sauces and soups. Egg rolls do in fact have egg in the wrappers, but vegetable spring rolls are usually vegan. Ma Po Tofu is usually prepared with ground pork in addition to the tofu, but many places will omit the pork if you ask. Also, oyster sauce is usually made with oysters (but you can find a mushroom version in Asian groceries if cooking for yourself). If you're lucky enough to find a Buddhist Chinese restaurant, you're set — they're almost all completely vegan and will have mock meats galore.

THAI, VIETNAMESE, AND OTHER SOUTHEAST ASIAN: We've had lots of luck with Thai restaurants because they also usually have a vegetarian section in their menus. You do need to ask about fish sauce in the curries or sauces in Southeast Asian restaurants — many places will be able to omit it if you ask, although some use pre-mixed sauces and therefore can't (or won't) leave it out of the dish. Also, the same warning from above applies about oyster sauce.

KOREAN AND JAPANESE: These two cuisines love to put fish in everything, so you have to be extra careful. Most Korean places are fairly non-vegan friendly, but you can sometimes find a tofu dish or two that doesn't have meat stock or fish in it, or you can get veggie bibimbap, which is rice and a bunch of vegetables on top with a spicy sauce (without the egg on top). At a Japanese restaurant, you'll find fish in the soup stock and egg in the tempura batter. We usually end up eating seaweed salad, edamame, and veggie sushi rolls (watch out for mayo — yes, seriously), but sometimes you can find tofu and other dishes that don't have fish or meat in them, or soups that use seaweed stock.

INDIAN AND SOUTH ASIAN: There's a ton to eat at Indian restaurants that's vegetarian — but unfortunately not vegan. Some of the non-vegan stuff is obvious from the menu description — milk, yogurt, cream, or cheese (paneer) — but otherwise it might be hidden in the dish in the form of ghee (clarified butter). You need to ask about ghee in every dish that appears to be vegan. Some places will be able to make the dishes without ghee, or can point you to others that contain oil instead. Also, naan is usually made with yogurt in the dough, and other breads might come slathered in butter.

ITALIAN: Again, another place where you're likely to find plenty of vegetarian options, but not so much that's outright vegan. But, more often than not, they can accommodate you by removing the cheese from a dish or by making you something special like pasta with oil, vegetables, and garlic. Ask about cheese or butter in the pizza dough, meat, meat stock, cheese, or butter in the sauce, cheese on top of salads and pasta, and egg in the pasta. (Fresh pasta is almost always made with egg, but dried pasta is usually vegan.) Also, things that are breaded and fried are often dipped in egg first. You might get weird looks by asking for a pizza without cheese and instead loaded with vegetables, but who cares. Cheeseless pizza is actually quite good (think of it as flatbread with roasted vegetables.)

ETHIOPIAN: If you ever get the chance to try Ethiopian cuisine, do so. The meals are served on a huge platter covered with a spongy bread called injera, with all the dishes placed in small piles on top. Everyone rips off some of the bread and scoops up the food with it, family style. You can get an all-vegan assortment of dishes that include spiced lentils, cabbage, greens, and other legumes and vegetables. You will leave absolutely stuffed. (Warning — the injera seems to expand in your stomach after you leave the restaurant, so you might sit around going "oh, I ate too much and I feel like I'm going to explode" for some time afterwards if you're not careful.)

MEXICAN: Your best and easiest bet at a Mexican or Tex-Mex restaurant is the veggie fajitas. Otherwise, you can often get a bean burrito or enchilada without the cheese and sour cream. Ask about meat stock in the rice and beans, dairy in the guacamole (grrr, which is just so wrong), and lard in the flour tortillas. You may have to remind them to keep the cheese off things.

MIDDLE EASTERN AND NORTHERN AFRICAN (MEDITERRANEAN):
Luckily, Middle Eastern and Mediterranean cuisines use a lot of olive oil instead of butter and have many vegan salads and things that you can eat with pita bread. Look for Lebanese, Israeli, Morrocan, and Egyptian food, where you'll find falafel, hummus, tabouli, baba ganoush, ful medames, couscous, and other tasty vegetable-based dishes and salads. Watch out for cheese and yogurt-based condiments and sauces.

Lastly, one way for you to be prepared and therefore hopefully enjoy yourself more is to use "The Google." If you know where you're going ahead of time, you can often find a menu for the restaurant online, and you may even be able to call ahead to ask questions. Or, you can search for vegan-friendly restaurants in one of the many dining guides that are out there written specifically for vegans and vegetarians, and grouped by city or area. Some of these are amalgamated sites like HappyCow, and others are city-specific. You can also use sites like MenuPages or Yelp to get restaurant reviews and information and search for vegetarian restaurants.

It's important to keep in mind that you can't expect the world to cater to you and to always be vegan-friendly. It's a non-vegan world, and most societies are set up to reify and perpetuate this fact. If you're upset about the lack of vegan options in restaurants, do something about it instead of just complaining! Educate people so there are more vegans in the world (see Chapters 2 and 6), get restaurants to understand that we should be catered to, and be nice to and thank the ones that do. Hey, if you're the entrepreneurial type, you can even start your own vegan restaurant or café!

On the Road Again

So you're all set for your cross-country road trip. iPod full? Check. Suitcases packed? Check. Enormous amounts of money saved up to pay for gas? Check. Vegan survival kit? Huh? If you've been on America's highways lately, you've noticed that there aren't exactly a lot of vegan-friendly choices out there right off the interstate.[11] But there are plenty of ways that you can make sure you don't go hungry when you're traveling, if you prepare ahead and if you know what to look for.

If at all possible, avoid fast food places like the plague. Not only are there very few options for vegans, but you're also supporting a horrible industry.[12] That said, sometimes you are desperately hungry, or you forgot to plan ahead and you need something to eat and there's nothing else available. There are two fast food places that have reliable vegan options: Subway and Taco Bell. At Subway, you can get a veggie delight on hearty Italian (the wheat bread has honey and most others have honey or cheese), and you can get oil, vinegar, mustard, or sweet onion sauce for a condiment. The veggie patty available at some Subways is not vegan. At Taco Bell, you can get a bean burrito (but ask for it without cheese and check before you take a bite to make sure it doesn't have cheese), veggie fajita wraps (without sour cream), rice, and salsa and guacamole.

To avoid having to go into a fast food restaurant, plan ahead, or consider other options. Self-catering at a grocery store can provide you with some healthier and heartier options than fast food places. Many supermarkets have a salad and fruit bar, some have elaborate take-out type food, and you can always grab sandwich ingredients, fresh fruit, cereal, or even canned beans if you can stand eating them right out of the can (and have a can opener, of course). The self-catering option works especially well when you're already at your destination — you can grab a bunch of things and take them back to your hotel room. You can heat up hot water in the room's coffee maker for oatmeal or instant soups, and even put a few essentials on ice if there's no refrigerator. (Gotta love the hotels with microwaves and mini-fridges — they've allowed us to eat pretty well in otherwise dire food circumstances.) Some friends of ours take a co-op directory with them when they travel (http://www.cooperativegrocer.coop/coops/) so they can search out good places to stop in addition to finding good eats at the co-op; their reasoning is that if a town has a co-op, it probably has other cool things as well.

The best way to make sure you will eat well on the road is to travel with your own vegan survival kit. For us, this usually includes a plethora of snacks, nuts, fruit, a sandwich, a thermos of coffee, packets of vegan coffee creamer (available online), small juice-box sized containers of soymilk, food in bar form, and perhaps something quick for breakfast. If we're in the car, we don't have to be forced to get black convenience store coffee that's been sitting around for hours and greasy potato chips, and if we've packed lunch, we can avoid fast food restaurants. This is also especially helpful if you're not sure what the food options are going to be like at your destination or if you won't have time to hunt down a grocery store. If you're traveling to a conference or business meetings, be sure to pack snacks to carry with you in your bag or briefcase for during the day, because it's often hard to escape the meeting site to find food. Having something you can eat for breakfast and/or something to get your coffee the way you like it is important as well. Breakfast can be the most difficult meal for vegan options when you're out and about, because only some places have soymilk (Starbucks, most reliably), and most of the food options you will find are loaded with eggs and dairy.

Plus, do you really want to go some place and have to smell eggs cooking? (Once you become vegan for a while, that becomes one of the most vile smells on the planet.) We usually end up eating fruit, granola, bars, or cereal (with soymilk that we put on ice the night before), but there are a lot of other options if you're creative. Not sure what to stock your vegan survival kit with? Check out Sarah Kramer's book *Vegan A Go-Go: A Cookbook and Survival Manual for Vegans on the Road* (which is conveniently travel-sized) for some tips on what to make before you go or once you get there. If you're interested in trying new and interesting vegan snacks, stock up at one of the online vegan stores as well.

The vegan survival kit can also help you when traveling by plane. Because of cutbacks, you have to be on a pretty long flight before the airlines will actually provide you with a meal. If you are lucky (or is it unlucky?) enough to have a meal on your flight, call the airline a few days in advance to request a vegan meal. Otherwise, you'll be glad you packed that bag of nuts, carrot sticks, dried fruit, and your favorite energy bar, and you just have to pray that you're not sitting next to someone who decided that it would be a good idea to bring a fast-food burger on the plane with them. Your vegan survival kit will also come in handy, as you'll inevitably be sitting around airports for long periods of time. You can even pack yourself a sandwich to eat at some point during your trip — nut butter and jelly travels well. Just don't pack any liquids or foods like soy yogurt since they won't make it past security. If you find yourself without your survival kit or you've already eaten everything and still need a bite to eat, it is actually fairly easy to find something that's vegan in the airport, especially in large airports. It may not be the healthiest food on the planet, but you can find something that will hold you over. On our travels, we've found everything from salads to bagels to seitan sandwiches (thank you, Chicago!) to vegan "chicken" Lo Mein (hooray, Boston!) and many different types of snacks. It may take some wandering around to different vendors, but what else are you going to do while you wait?

If you're off to an international destination where you don't speak the language, find out how to say "I'm vegan" (although there's not always an exact equivalent — strict vegetarian might work better), and learn how to ask basic questions like "does it have milk, meat, chicken, fish, eggs?" or "I don't eat milk, meat, chicken, fish, eggs, cheese, etc." Knowing the words for meat, chicken, fish, and eggs are important, because around the world the term "meat" often only covers four-legged creatures, not birds or fish. The International Vegetarian Union (http://www.ivu.org) has a list of handy phrases in many languages, as well as a database where you can search for information on hotels and vegan-friendly restaurants around the world. When you're abroad, look for open-air markets that may have wonderful and inexpensive produce to try. Research the local cuisine ahead of time if you can, so you know what kinds of things to look for and expect in restaurants. If you're ever stuck, you can always try to find a Chinese restaurant or a Govinda, which are prevalent all around the world and have options for vegans. And just a reminder — just because you are traveling to another culture does not mean that you have to eat whatever animal product that is their local delicacy to really "experience" that culture. Similarly, just because you don't feel like looking for vegan food when in a strange place does not make it okay to have that piece of cheese or that meat dish. If you believe that animal cruelty is wrong, then you shouldn't participate in it on purpose to fill your belly, ever.

Planning ahead when you travel can make your experience much more enjoyable and much more stress-free. Remember that no one else is going to take care of you, so you need to do your research, pack some snacks and other supplies, and be prepared to ask questions. If you do, you can spend much more time enjoying your destination, and much less time wandering around aimlessly looking for food.

Don't Be Grumpy (Abundance, Not Deprivation Revisited)

It's easy to be a vegan even in what might seem to be a very non-vegan place if you know what to look for, how to cook, what questions to ask, and if you have the right attitude. It might take you some time to get used to reading labels, finding the brands that have vegan options, figuring out where to dine, and what to make for dinner (and accidents happen to the best of us), but it gets much easier the longer you're vegan, and even becomes second-nature. In case you haven't noticed from this chapter, GIYF (Google is your friend). There's tons of information out there on the Internet from your fellow vegans that can also help you along your way, lots of vegan recipes to try, and plenty of places to find vegan foods that you might not be able to get locally.

Being miserable, feeling deprived, or being generally grumpy isn't going to help anyone, especially yourself. Feel empowered by your choice to become vegan. The non-vegans in the world might think you are a freak, but they're the ones who think it's okay to eat dead animals and to enslave animals to produce milk and eggs. Be happy and confident as you go into that restaurant to ask your questions, as you walk your cart around the grocery store and check out the labels, and as you cook your cruelty-free meal with antioxidant-filled vegetables. If the non-vegan world is frustrating you or getting you down, then see Chapters 2 and 6 for tips on how to do something about it.

Notes to Chapter 4

1   Although, thinking about food in this way will make you want to smack the first person who says to you "oh, right, sorry, you can't have that piece of cake because you're vegan." Although you may want to shout back "No, I don't want to eat your pus-filled cow secretions and chicken menstrual products!" and knock the table over and run out of the room, restrain yourself and say something polite like "yeah, no thanks."

2   This is especially helpful if you previously liked to smother things in cheese.

3   Damn you, dirty hippies!

4   Some people find soymilk to have an aftertaste when they first try it. Give it time, and you won't notice it any more. Or, try one of the many other cows' milk alternatives mentioned.

5   http://www.wnd.com/news/article.asp?ARTICLE_ID=53327 and http://counterknowledge.com/2008/08/eat-soy-and-youre-gay/.

6   Actually, starving your children will kill them, not feeding them a proper vegan diet: http://www.11alive.com/news/article_news.aspx?storyid=96364.

7   Joel Fuhrman, *Eat For Health: Lose Weight, Keep It Off, Look Younger, Live Longer* (Flemington, NJ: Gift of Health Press, 2008).

8   If you're ever bored and you feel like watching vegans attack one another mindlessly, pop on over to a vegan forum and put up a post titled "IS HONEY VEGAN?" (Yeah, in all caps, they'll love you even more for that). We're obviously kidding, please don't do this. You'll just be a pedantic pain in the ass.

9   If you'd like to learn more about bees, read up on them in wikipedia. They're quite fascinating insects — they even do their own little dance!

10   Despite the name, lactic acid, found in jars of olives, pickles, and the like, is usually plant-derived.

11   And people from other countries such as Australia inform us that the same is true elsewhere.

12   You can probably guess the many reasons why the fast food industry is so horrible, but for a thorough investigation into the suffering behind the convenience, we recommend that you read *Fast Food Nation* by Eric Schlosser.

CHAPTER 5

IT'S NOT JUST ABOUT FOOD

IF YOU'VE MADE IT THIS FAR INTO THE BOOK, it should come as no surprise to you that veganism goes far beyond what you put in your mouth — it is about eliminating the use of animal products in the whole of your life where possible as a living protest against animal exploitation. So, this could include what you wear, what you clean yourself and your living space with, what you put on your face and hair to make yourself look pretty, and even what you use to get it on. (What could possibly be not vegan about sex, you ask? You'd be surprised. Read on.)

As we said in Chapter 1, however, the primary motivation for veganism is not personal purity; you cannot avoid every single animal product living in today's society because sometimes there is no alternative. Do you drive or ride a bike or take the bus? There are animal products in the tires. Do you walk? You're likely to unwittingly step on an insect at some point in your travels. Don't let any of this discourage you or let it be an excuse to do nothing because there's no completely perfect 100 percent pure solution. There are plenty of areas in your life in which you do have a choice as to what to buy, make, or use, and you can easily choose the compassionate (i.e. vegan) route if you know what to look for and where to look.

In the most basic terms, there's no need to wear anything that is made out of leather, wool, feathers, down, bone, pearl, silk, shell, or fur since there are plenty of vegan alternatives out there to clothe yourself with. Things like leather and fur are obviously not vegan, since you have to kill the animal to get them. But as with dairy, many people think that products such as wool aren't a big deal because it's "sustainable"[1] and you don't have to kill the animal to get it, right? It's just like giving the sheep a pleasant little haircut, isn't it? Well, just like with the cows who produce dairy products, there's no idyllic pasture that the sheep go to when they get old. When they are no longer useful, they are killed. And as you might suspect, the sheep aren't treated particularly nicely either. They are castrated without anesthetic, their tails are docked, and many are subjected to a procedure called mulesing,[2] during which a strip of the skin on their hindquarters is removed to prevent fly and maggot infestation (which is common in the sheep that are bred to have extra skin and thus extra wool). But even if the sheep were fed the finest of grasses, massaged and given mani-pedis every day before being killed in the most gentle of manners, that would still be no excuse to buy wool. Using wool reifies the notion that using animal products is an acceptable means to an end, and this attitude and approach to the status of animals has locked them into a position of subordination for millennia.

Because you don't need to wear any animal product to survive, there's no need to do so, even if you are a major fashionista and think you might die without the latest Prada bag or Manolo Blahnik shoes. Through your wardrobe you can send the message that animals are not things to be exploited for fashion. You might know plenty of vegetarians who wear leather and have no problem with it, and you yourself might not think it's as bad as eating animals, because you figure the animal was already killed for some other purpose. Or, you might think that buying second-hand, non-vegan items from a thrift store is okay because you aren't creating demand for the item, and you want to make sure it doesn't go to waste by being thrown away before it's worn out. But think about it — any time you are out in the world wearing leather shoes or a wool sweater, you are a walking contradiction, sending the wrong message about veganism and your commitment to it. Wearing leather or wool or other animal products as an ethical vegan is every bit as confusing as being a feminist who argues for the objectification of women as mere sexual objects, and not as whole, full human beings.

Additionally, even though it is nowhere near fair, as a vegan you are going to represent all of vegandom every time you interact with someone else, and they are going to look for hypocrisy and contradiction so they can have a glimmer of hope that being vegan is just too hard and not possible. In fact, you will most likely get scanned for any obvious animal products you are wearing when you mention you are vegan to someone who would love to see you slip up — just watch for the eyes going to your shoes, your belt, and your coat. Though you obviously want to avoid the "gotchas" of some-one being able to point out the contradictions, you also can't possibly ever hope to make the case against animal exploita-tion if you're wearing the skin of a dead animal, no matter where you bought it or why you have it.

But What Do I Do With the Old Leather?

This brings us to the sticky situation of having decided to go vegan and then wondering what to do with all the leather, wool, and down items that you have in your closet. It's a little more complicated than getting rid of the non-vegan food in your refrigerator, because you most likely only had a week or two worth of items to eat anyway. But you were probably hoping those leather boots you bought last month would last a few years, and perhaps you were lamenting the fact that your down comforter was so expensive and still is nowhere near worn out. When we first went vegan, were surprised by the number of non-vegan items we had in our closet and in our home — probably made worse by the fact that we lived somewhere where it routinely went below 0° F during the winters and we decided to dress like arctic explorers in huge down coats to stay warm. (Seriously, you should have seen the size of Bob's winter coat — it looked like the ones you see on the Discovery channel worn by the guys scaling Everest.)

Unfortunately, the vast majority of us can't afford to go out and buy ourselves and entire new wardrobe in one day. (If you can, problem solved! Go out and buy yourself a new vegan wardrobe immediately.) There are basically two options you have for your "pregan" (pre-vegan) items: you can either use them until they wear out, or you can give them away or sell them. The first option may seem okay at first, but it presents some problems in practice. After you've been vegan for some time, wearing leather and wool can seem downright morbid, because you find yourself thinking about where it came from. Additionally, there's the problem we just mentioned above of seeming contradictory or hypocritical even though you don't want to be. You can explain to people that you recently went vegan and you're waiting until the shoes wear out, but that gets tiresome after awhile.

Giving the items away or selling them is your best bet if you can manage it. If you can't do it all at once, do it piecemeal. Start with the most obviously non-vegan things like the shoes you wear all the time out of the house and leather coats, or things that aren't quite as expensive to replace, like belts. Give them to the local thrift store or Goodwill, or if they're in great shape, sell them on eBay or Craigslist. Then little by little start getting rid of your other, less obvious or more expensive items, like your pillow and comforter or down or wool coat, or the dress shoes you wear once a year. If you're holding onto things for sentimental reasons, then keep the item and put it away in a special spot somewhere where you can take it out once in awhile and think of grandma or your favorite summer at the beach.

Pleather is Punk

Okay, so you've gotten rid of your favorite pair of leather shoes and your down coat. Now what? Where do you find replacements? Is there life after leather? Will you be forced to wear cheap leather knock-offs for the rest of your life? Luckily, there are alternatives to buying the skin of another animal for all budgets and fashion senses. If you live in places like New York City, San Diego, or Atlanta, you will be lucky enough to shop in person at an all-vegan store.[3] Otherwise, you'll either have to shop online or scour the "regular" stores for vegan goods.

Thankfully, the Internet has come to the rescue for many vegans who can't find anything but Crocs, flip-flops, and non-ironic 80s-style jean jackets locally. Many of the online vegan stores mentioned in the food chapter also carry shoes and some clothing, and you can find even more at places like MooShoes, Alternative Outfitters, VeganWares (Australia), Vegetarian Shoes (UK), and the like — just Google vegan shoes, vegan bags, or vegan clothing. In addition, you can find many choices at places like Zappos or even Amazon, and get blazingly fast shipping. (Although we recommend browsing the all-vegan or small retailers first, since it's always good to support the small businesses that are trying to make a go of it and who share your ethical concerns.)

In real life, you can find vegan shoes at most retail stores — just look for the words "All Man-Made Materials." (And like the vegan in the grocery store finding bread with no honey or whey, you'll find the fellow vegan doing a happy dance upon spotting the man-made label.) Payless has many options if you're looking to find things on a budget, and even some high-end retailers have one or two vegan options as well.

In fact, there are vegan versions of all your must-have types of shoes including sandals, four-inch pumps, hiking boots, and running shoes (in fact, most actual running shoes are vegan, although other types of workout or sport shoes may not be). Some of the more expensive vegan shoes use materials that are much stronger than the cheap vegan shoes, so they do tend to last longer. Some materials also look a lot like leather, which can be a good or a bad thing, depending on your opinion. Some people want to get away from the look of leather because it creates a new sense of what's fashionable, rather than trying to look like dead cow. Others like to make a statement that you can have the look of leather without killing anything. Bob, for example, loves his 14-hole steel-toed pleather boots, because they simply kick ass. Plus, when people inevitably point at you and say "Yeah, but your boots are leatherrrrrrr!!!!!" you can show them that they really aren't. Bob has had to go as far as holding up the sole of the shoe — imprinted with the words VEGETARIAN SHOES — to people's faces to prove his point.

Replacing down and wool can be fairly easy since cotton and synthetic fibers abound, and you can easily read the labels on clothing and items like pillows, comforters, and rugs. There are a few exceptions where it may be difficult — dressy winter coats and coats rated for extreme cold, and suits. There are some alternatives to dressy winter coats, but most of them are only suitable for more mild winters. If you live where it is ridiculously, cruelly cold (like we used to), you may need to layer fairly extensively if you use one of these synthetic dressy coats, or only wear them when it's not quite as cold. Many parka-type coats that can keep you toasty when the wind chill is -30° F tend to be down — after all, down is very warm, that's why geese and ducks need it! But, thanks to modern science, we now have amazing synthetic materials such as PrimaLoft or fleece (not wool fleece, but Polartec fleece) that do a pretty good job without the downsides of cotton (i.e. when it gets wet it is useless to keep you warm). It is pretty easy these days to find coats with one of these materials as the primary fill material or with a layer of it. Plus, if you can always add a layer of fleece if you find yourself getting too chilly. (Or, you can move somewhere warmer, which we highly suggest for the mental health value.) As for suits, the challenge isn't necessarily finding vegan versions — there are plenty of polyester suits out there — it's finding ones you would want to wear in public without breaking the bank for some designer label, and finding ones you would want to wear in the winter without freezing. You may just have to scour the stores for something that suits you. (Ha, get it! Suits you. Sorry, yet another bad pun.)

If, unlike us, you are extremely resourceful, you can even make your own clothing and accessories. In fact, there's a whole group on Etsy.com dedicated to other people's hand-made vegan items, which is another great resource if you're looking for an awesome hat, scarf, bag, jewelry, art, and more. Another alternative to mainstream shopping is thrift stores, especially if you have a keen eye and provided that you get there before all the hipsters do. Sarah Kramer of govegan.net is a big fan and proponent of the thrift store and vintage ethic, so if you want to know more, go to her site or pick up one of her books. Like we said above, though, buying some-thing second-hand is not an excuse to buy leather, wool, or any other animal product. It still presents the animal product as a legitimate form of animal use, which it is not. Leave the leather and wool for someone else to buy, and snatch up all the great vegan items.

Lastly, some of you may be wondering about some required items that you have to wear for work that may not be vegan. We know of many people who, for instance, are mandated by law to wear a certain type of safety boot to work, and they don't come in non-vegan versions. Others may have to wear wool or leather as part of a uniform. In most cases, you don't have much of a choice, and therefore must wear the non-vegan item. Remember, it's about being vegan when possible, and this may not be one of those times. Sometimes, depending on the circumstances, you may be able to convince your bosses or organization to let you wear a vegan version of the uniform or required clothing. You need to be able to read the situation to figure out whether or not this is possible, but it may be if you are willing to ask. We know of one actress who called into our podcast who was originally required to wear a fur stole for her role, but she convinced those in charge of the play to let her get a nice faux fur instead, and all parties ended up happy.

It may seem like a pain at first to find vegan clothing and accessories and to replace what you already have. Believe us, we know how frustrating it can be when you're looking for a non-wool sweater and it seems like everything you find has angora, wool, or cashmere in the label[4]. But in time you start to learn about places where you can consistently find items you like, and it gets easier. (Remember, like we said in Chapter 4 — Google is Your Friend if you need to find vegan items on the Internet.) Who knows — maybe you'll be inspired to design an all-vegan clothing line or start your own vegan store (any fashion designers out there?). In the end, you'll find that you'll walk taller in your new vegan gear. It gives you confidence and a sense of well being to know that no animals were killed for your fashion.

Vegan Cosmetics, Toiletries, and Cleaning Supplies

Animal products have a tendency to show up in places where we least expect them, and in things that we rely on every day: soap, deodorant, medicines, makeup, lip balm, toothpaste, shaving cream, lotion, and many other drugstore items. Animal ingredients are cheap and plentiful, and are used without question by many large companies who also test their products on animals. These ingredients are also harder to identify than the dairy and egg-derivatives in grocery items, since many are only listed by their chemical name. You might think that searching the ingredient list of not only your groceries but also your toiletries is a major pain in the ass. Perhaps you'll conclude after skimming enough ingredient lists that this level of vigilance is unnecessary, but we'd like to convince you that the situation is not as bad as it sounds. Since there are so many non-animal alternatives, it is relatively easy to find products that are vegan-friendly and cruelty-free. And after you learn about the process used to get animal products into most cosmetics and toiletries, you'll probably want to seek out animal-free options anyway.

Learning about the rendering process is essential for understanding why it is necessary for vegans to be concerned about what's in the products they use. Once animals are slaughtered, all the leftover parts (bones, ligaments, hooves, brains, spinal columns, eyeballs, intestines, and other random parts that aren't being eaten by foodies somewhere) are sent off to a rendering plant, along with animals from the slaughterhouse dead pile (ones that died before making it to slaughter), euthanized animals from shelters and zoos, horses, road kill, and expired meat from grocery store. (We're not making this up.[5]) The bones, fats, and proteins are all separated, and then made into various products. Remember the gelatin in Jell-O, marshmallows, and candies (in addition to some gel capsules and film) we mentioned in Chapter 4? That's where it comes from. The protein bits get fed to your companion animals, most likely, and are also often fed back to livestock in what often becomes a strange form of cannibalism (ever wonder where mad cow came from?). Other bits, especially the fats, get made into cosmetics, soaps, shaving cream, shampoo, crayons, candles, dryer sheets, and fabric softener. Pretty disgusting, isn't it? Now, do you really want to be brushing your teeth with that, or be cleaning yourself with it?

Luckily, there are many non-animal-based equivalents to the things that come out of the rendering process. Unfortunately, animal-based products are cheap and readily available because of the billions of animals slaughtered every year. In addition, getting every last bit of money possible out of every animal is necessary to make a profit in the animal industry. It's a huge business, and therefore these products show up in just about every product imaginable in your local drug store or grocery store.

The best way to find out about insidious animal ingredients is to get a copy of a book like *Animal Ingredients A to Z*, find an online or iPod version of a list, or research the ingredients online. These books/lists are extremely useful to have around or take with you when you shop.

Some of the more common ingredients you'll run into include:

GLYCERIN: usually made out of animal fats left after making soaps. Ever see *Fight Club*? Same principle applies here. Glycerin shows up in lotions, shampoos and conditioners, soaps and body washes, cosmetics, tattoo ink, and toothpaste. It is particularly annoying, because there is a plant-based form of glycerin, so just by looking at the label you have no idea what the source is unless the company is nice enough to put plant-based after it. The only way to be completely sure is to contact the manufacturer, though chances are that most mainstream (read: made by big company that probably tests on animals anyway) products use animal-based glycerin.

LANOLIN: comes from sheep's wool and is found in many lotions and body washes, as well as lip balm and other skin-care products. Vegetable oils can serve a similar function without harming sheep.

STEARIC ACID (AND OTHER DERIVATIVES WITH THE PREFIX STEARO-): another rendering product found in shaving cream, cosmetics, hairspray, and even some food and chewing gum. You can get stearic acid from plants (like coconuts, for instance), but more often than not it's the animal-derived version in most mainstream products.

There are sadly many other insidious by-products of rendering found in various toiletries and cleaning products, including the already mentioned gelatin, beeswax and honey, polysorbates, alpha-hydroxy acid, keratin and other proteins, silk, and tallow (a fat used in dryer sheets and fabric softeners to make your clothes feel soft and have less static).

If you're ever not sure about whether the glycerin or stearic acid or the like in your favorite products is animal or plant derived, call or write the company that manufactures it, or look online to see if anyone else has already done the research for you. That way you'll be sure you know the source, and you'll also be letting the company know that there are people out there who don't want to buy their product if it has animal bits in it.

At this point you're probably wondering how you can avoid all of these ingredients if they're so very common and in most mainstream products. Luckily, there are many vegan-friendly brands to look for that can be found in some well-stocked drug and grocery stores, health food stores and co-ops, specialty stores or salons, and online: Alba, Aubrey Organics, Aveda, Beauty Without Cruelty, Giovanni, JASON, Kiss My Face, and Lush just to name a few. Please be aware that not all products from these companies are vegan — they do use lanolin, beeswax or honey, and/or carmine in some of their products — but chances are that the ones that are vegan are labeled as such or it is easy to tell from the label. If you don't feel like reading the labels, you can always shop at one of the all-vegan online stores, where they do the label reading for you (and you're also supporting fellow vegans!).

You'll notice that many of the products from these companies are promoted as eco-friendly and cruelty-free — and in fact, if you search out those types of products, chances are that you'll find at least some vegan items that weren't tested on animals. Not all eco-friendly and "cruelty-free" products are vegan, though, so be on the look-out for those products that are labeled as not being tested on animals but that contain animal by-products. (No, it doesn't make sense. They don't want to harm the animals to test the products, but they'll kill animals and use their parts for their ingredients? Go figure.) The same goes for products used for cleaning your house — you can find many vegan items in the eco-friendly aisle from brands such as Method (all their products are 100 percent vegan and found in the US, UK, and Canada), Ecover, Seventh Generation, or Mrs. Meyer's Clean Day. Plus, it's nice to not have to use so many deadly chemicals both for your health as well as the health of your family and companion animals.

You'll also notice that these products tend to be a little more expensive than most mainstream products. What we've found, however, is that these products tend to last longer because they are of higher quality, and so you break even or sometimes save money over the long run (and sometimes you can find deals at places like Trader Joe's or discount stores too). If you're hurting for cash, like to make things yourself, or just really want to be sure that your products are vegan, you can always make your own beauty and cleaning products. It's really quite amazing what you can do with baking soda, vinegar, and salt.[6]

The goal with beauty and cleaning products is to reduce your reliance on animal-based products when you can, though you may find that it is impossible to be 100 percent animal free in this arena. If you accidentally buy a product that you later find out to have an animal ingredient in it, return it if you haven't used it or give it away and learn from your newfound knowledge and buy something else next time.

Medications

Although we discussed this topic in Chapter 1, we need to reiterate here the issue of animal products in medications, especially prescription meds. Many people have asked us if they should take their prescription medication even though they know it has animal products in it. OF COURSE YOU SHOULD. Here's the thing about medications. At least in the United States, all of them are required by law to be tested on animals before being approved and going to market, and there's no way around this. In addition, the vast majority of them contain some animal-derived ingredient or another. Regardless, it is absolutely ridiculous to suggest that you should not take a medication, especially one that you absolutely need or that your doctor told you to take, just because the medications are not vegan. We're not just saying this so we don't get in trouble. We really believe that this is one of those situations in which you are not able to take the vegan route and therefore you must take the non-vegan route. If you don't take your medications, you at the very least suffer, and at the most could do long-term damage to your health or worse. It is not worth it. Many people will also not take over-the-counter meds or birth control pills because they are not vegan; again, you are not obligated to suffer in this instance by not taking the medications, because you have no choice but to participate in the system as it is.[7] If you are unhealthy, not only do you not do yourself any favors, you also do veganism no favors. (If you remain confused about our point on medications, please refer back to the hypothetical that we quote from Gary Francione in Chapter 1; this analogy helps to clear things up.)

One place you do have a choice of a vegan alternative is with over-the-counter supplements, such as vitamins and herbs. Many are packaged with gelatin capsules, but you can find ones with vegan capsules in many health food stores and online. In addition, you can find vegan versions of things like Vitamin D, Omega-3s, Glucosamine, etc. instead of having to rely on fish oil or other animal products.

If you're upset by the state of affairs with regard to medication, instead of not taking your pills, try to get more people to go vegan or educate people on the state of animal testing[8] so that there will be more awareness of these issues and less demand for the use of animal testing overall.

Don't Read This Section If You're Under 18

Titling any section like that virtually guarantees that those under 18 will read it, but what can we do? Were Bob under 18 and not one of the authors of this book, this section would probably be the first thing that he'd have read. Anyway, in this section, we talk about yet one more aspect of personal care: sex. We're going to talk about stuff that deals with nasty, dirty, fun things and how to keep doing your dirty, nasty, fun things without harming animals in the process. If talk of sex bothers you, stop being such a prude. (Ah, we're just kidding.) Seriously, though, if you have delicate sensibilities or you're a young'un, just flip to the next section.

Okay, with that said and out of the way, don't say we didn't warn you.

CONDOMS AND SAFE SEX SUPPLIES

At the beginning of the chapter we posed the question 'what could possibly be not vegan about getting it on?' Well, most condoms, for one. Shockingly, many latex condoms are produced using casein (the same milk protein found in "vegetarian" cheeses and other "non-dairy" products we mentioned in Chapter 4). This is of course a gigantic pain in the ass, but the good news is that there are condoms out there that contain no animal products and are not tested on animals. Glyde, an Australian company, makes vegan latex condoms, dams, and gloves in a number of sizes and flavors. We've personally never seen them in any local store, but they are easy to find online at the all-vegan stores. Order a bunch to have around for when you need them! (But of course, pay attention to the expiration date, and never keep them stored in a wallet, since they tend to weaken from the heat and the pressure of being sandwiched between your butt cheek and whatever your butt cheek is resting on.) Another vegan brand, Condomi condoms, are widely available in Europe but not available in the US.

OTHER FUN THINGS: LUBE, TOYS, AND PLEATHER

If you're using latex condoms and want some lube, you should always use a water-based lube since oil-based ones can reduce the efficacy of the condoms. Like many other manufactured health products, lubes can contain animal by-products, usually glycerin. Fortunately, there are plenty of vegan lubes on the market that either have plant-sourced glycerin and other ingredients, or no glycerin at all (because some people's skin gets irritated by it). Check out different brands to see what you like online at places like Babeland or The Sensual Vegan.

Babeland and The Sensual Vegan also carry a wide range of sex toys (Babeland carries vegan and non-vegan items, but they are very good about labeling most things that are vegan.) The nice part about both of these sites is that they're generally sex-positive and they're discreet. Because of non-descript labeling and packaging that a company like Babeland uses, you can order confident in the knowledge that a box will not arrive at your doorstep with "YOUR HUGE DILDO ORDER" emblazoned on the side in 150-point Impact. And speaking of huge dildo orders, most silicone sex toys are vegan, and silicone is the best material for sex toys anyway. The downside is that silicone toys aren't cheap, but they're worth the money because they're durable, easy to clean, and don't hold odors. The ones you need to watch out for are "jelly rubber" items that contain mystery ingredients, so you cannot be sure that they're animal-free unless the manufacturer explicitly says they are. (And some of these items may also contain relatively toxic chemicals like phthalates that you probably don't want to be putting anywhere in the immediate vicinity of your nether-regions, either.)

But what is the vegan leather fetishist to do? Seriously, if you're into leather products but you abhor the cruelty involved in making them, you can now find vegan substitutes for most of your leather and BDSM needs. Again, Babeland has some vegan dildo harnesses, and Vegan Erotica has fake leather products that have the look, feel, and durability of the real thing. You can get spiked collars, belts, harnesses, restraints, and hitting toys that are made with a product called Lorica, which according to the Vegan Erotica website is a synthetic leather that is permeable to water vapor, is water repellent, machine washable, and resistant to tearing, splitting, and scratching.

Whatever kinds of fun, interesting, weird, or just plain kinky stuff you're into, odds are good that you can find a vegan or animal-friendly way of expressing your desires; you may just have to resort to the Internet to get what you need, yet again.

TATTOOING

There's simply no easy way to segue from sex toys into tattoos, so we're not even going to try. We thought before we closed out this chapter we'd briefly touch on tattooing and its implications for veganism. We both have large tattoo work, and will be most likely getting even more in the future. If you haven't had a tattoo, yeah, they hurt (but not so bad). For some reason, tattooing is addictive. You might begin by thinking that you're only going to get one, and then a few years later, you could end up with your arms or back covered. It really surprises you, but if you have one tattoo, you'll probably want another.

The problem for vegans and tattoos comes in the ink. Most inks use glycerin as a carrier, and this glycerin is most often animal-based. Still, there are ways around this. If you know a good tattoo artist, odds are that you can ask him or her to get vegan ink for you in advance of an appointment, which will probably cost you extra. You may also be able to find vegan tattoo shops, but these are far and few between. In the end, it is up to you to decide how big a deal vegan tattoo ink is.

BECAUSE ANIMAL EXPLOITATION GOES BEYOND animals being killed for food, ethical veganism also goes further than simply eliminating animal products from one's diet. Like other aspects of veganism, it can sometimes be challenging at first to make compassionate choices in a world that is structured around so much oppression. At times, it can be frustrating. You may feel that by eschewing leather, wool, down, and silk — on top of everything else — that you're the only person who cares about the plight of animals. This couldn't be further from the truth. If nothing else, this chapter shows that there are dedicated people who are promoting the abolition of animal slavery and exploitation through the development of vegan products, even in areas as diverse as sex toys and cosmetics. It might require a little extra planning and forethought, but before long, like other aspects of veganism, it becomes second nature. Best of all, it is completely worth it.

Notes to Chapter 5

1   We recently heard someone on a show about "green" houses calling wool rugs environmentally friendly because they are "sustainable." We think the sheep might disagree.

2   http://en.wikipedia.org/wiki/Mulesing

3   In NYC, you can even plunk down several hundred dollars in person to buy a pair of shoes from Natalie Portman's vegan line if you want.

4   Seriously — like who thought it was a good idea to make a sweater out of rabbits? And why do they make sweaters with 12 percent wool and the rest synthetic? It's a plot to annoy the vegans!

5   Howard Lyman, *Mad Cowboy: The Plain Truth From the Cattle Rancher Who Won't Eat Meat* (New York: Touchstone, 1998).

6   The cookbooks *How It All Vegan* and *The Garden of Vegan* by Sarah Kramer and Tanya Barnard have sections in them on creating your own cleaning and beauty supplies that are easy and cheap to make.

7   See Gary Francione reference in Chapter 1 p. 49.

8   A good online resource is pcrm.org, a group that promotes alternatives to medical animal testing, as well as the book *Sacred Cows and Golden Geese: The Human Cost of Experiments on Animals* by Jean Swingle Greek.

CHAPTER 6

GO VEGAN, STAY VEGAN

IT'S TIME.

It's time to dispense with the excuses, to own up to what is right, and to finally, once and for all, go vegan and stay vegan. By nature of the privilege you enjoy as a human, you could continue living as you have, eating animal products, and participating in these horrible cycles of violence. You could continue to indulge yourself, to convince yourself that it is too hard, or too radical, or too expensive, or too alienating. You could continue to be part of the problem and not part of the solution. Obviously, doing nothing is easier, and easy solutions are attractive, but easy solutions are not always solutions. When you look back on your life in a few decades, will you be happy with yourself if you were the person who knew about injustice and had the power to begin to change it, but who did nothing because it was too hard? Wouldn't you rather be the person who lived a life of principled conviction, and who made the right choices even though they were not always the easy ones?

Now is the time to cut off your participation in this insane system that kills billions upon billions of animals a year: going vegan is the way to do it. Veganism is the only logically and morally consistent choice in a world where killing and eating animals is normal. Eating "free-range," or "organic," or "local," or "humanely-raised," is no solution; it is your further entrenching the problem because you cannot be honest with yourself about the violence your choices are inflicting on others. Unlike most other people out there, we won't coddle you by telling you that half-measures are better than nothing. We won't make you feel warm and cuddly inside because you've "cut back" on eating animal products. We won't let you get away with the self-pitying excuses about you being compassionate to yourself as some justification for eating animal products. Instead, we ask you to be honest with yourself as an adult, to think critically and carefully about what you are doing, and to own up to your beliefs if you are serious about them. The world can never change for the better if people will not go about living their lives as conscious, thinking, and engaged members of the societies in which they live. If you're serious about according animals the value they deserve as the beings that they are in and of themselves, for themselves, you must go vegan. Otherwise, every single time you eat any animal product, you are undermining the interests of animals by silently reproducing the system that condemns billions of them to death year after year. If you are not vegan, you are part of the problem, and not part of the solution.

Going vegan is a statement with tremendous symbolic import, because every time you eat as a vegan you are choosing not to live as a speciesist. Simultaneously, you say to yourself and the others around you that things are not right as they are. You're taking a stance, living in the world powerfully and consciously, and showing others that animals need not suffer and die so that we can live. This will probably come as a big change in your life if you're not vegan yet, and so living as a new vegan can feel both empowering and overwhelming. You know you are doing the right thing and you feel good about making the ethical choice, but at the same time, you worry about feeling lonely or being the freak, you are saddened or angered by all the horrible things that happen to animals on a daily basis, and you may be freaked out by all the changes that you are going to have to make. If you feel this way, recognize that you are not alone. Many millions before you have made this change, and if we have our way, many millions more will continue to go vegan now and well into the future.

There are plenty of times that being vegan will feel frustrating, or times during which people will annoy you with their stupid questions and taunts. One way to stay mentally healthy through this is to harness the part of you that is empowered by going vegan and use it to make yourself a confident, proud vegan. Throughout the book, we've emphasized that you should be a good example of a happy, healthy vegan. We didn't repeat this point just because we felt like it. Aside from wanting you to remember the reasons you should be happy with your decision, we have found from experience that being happy, healthy, and confident in your veganism is really is the best way to get others to start thinking. By setting this example, you're showing people that it's not hard, that you're not deprived, and that veganism is entirely possible even in a very non-vegan world.

If you've done it for the right reasons, you should feel good about the commitment that you've made to go vegan. It is a positive and powerful step, and you are lending your voice to a cause that needs many more voices. As we said in Chapter 2, for veganism to be effective, it needs to grow into a movement of vegans dedicated to the abolition of animal exploitation. Most concretely, this means that we have to get others to go vegan, too. We're not asking you to stand on the street corner and shout at everyone walking by about the horrors they cause every day, nor are we asking that you go protest the circus or some other cause du jour is. All we ask is that as a vegan, you use your talents and energies to educate others about what veganism is, why it matters, and how it is the practical expression of the animal rights ethic.

You don't need a powerful organization behind you to do this, nor do you need millions of dollars or tons of time. The easiest thing to do is to not be afraid to call yourself a vegan, and to talk to other people when they have well-intentioned, curious questions about veganism. Beyond this, use your strengths and interests. If you like to cook, have friends over for a vegan meal, and shock the hell out of them by making it the best thing they've ever eaten. If you like to write, start a blog or write a pamphlet. If you like to talk to others, arrange a place where you can give a talk, have one-on-one discussions, or screen an AR-related film. If you can knit or sew, show people you can do so without animal fibers, or make your own items with vegan messages. If you're an artist, use your talents to make a statement in whatever media you use. If you are one of the many people who complains to us that they have no talent that is applicable to the cause — an assertion which we refuse to believe, by the way — volunteer to clean cages at a no-kill shelter, offer to peel potatoes for people cooking for events, give people rides to events, work on clean-up duty, lift stuff, or do something that requires no particular skill. Obviously we could go on and on. The point is, you can find ways to get the word out that send a positive message about veganism. You know how to reach the people around you the best, and you should think about how you can craft a message that will be best received by people to whom you can get the message. In thinking about who you might reach, remember that a great many people love animals, but that many of those people may not have made any real connections between the animals they love and the food they eat. Or, perhaps people have thought it through a little, but decided against veganism because they thought it was too hard, or they never really figured it was necessary, especially with all that "happy" free-range meat out there. You may have even been one of these people at some point. Certainly, we were. The thing to remember is that changing the world takes time. People are complex creatures, and many people are wary of making big changes in their lives, so don't get discouraged if you start doing this kind of work and no one goes vegan on the spot. For what it might be worth, on-the-spot "conversions" are pretty rare. Instead, you need to think of what you are doing as work that increases awareness and plants seeds. If you can get a few people to think critically about the issues, they may well walk away from their interaction with you and continue to ruminate on the issues. Some of the people you talk to will go vegan, and many won't. But you have to have the essential optimism of farmers the world over — the optimism that at least a few of your planted seeds will sprout.

We live in a world gone mad. As vegans, our refusal of the madness makes us the freaks. Yet, instead of running from the freakdom, you should embrace it. Your freakdom is you living your life not as someone who is simply content to do what society says because it is the way it has always been, but as someone who is living life with full awareness and consciousness. In this time of exceptional cowardice, your bravery will be an example to others, showing not only that people can change, but also that change is necessary. Being the lone voice of dissent is never easy, but the only people who have ever changed anything are those who have had the strength to stand up and say enough when presented with injustice.

Now is your time to stand up and object. Go vegan, and stay vegan.

INDEX

ABOUT TOFU HOUND PRESS

Tofu Hound Press is a small independent publisher with a commitment to publishing quality books on veganism, vegan cooking, animal rights, and related issues. We're small, but we have a lot of heart, and we work hard to bring valuable, vital, entertaining, and useful titles to market. Our goal is to publish smaller runs of books that otherwise might not make it to market through conventional publishers. We're just a few like-minded folks who want to get important ideas out there that might not see the light of day because of their limited profitability. For us profitable ideas aren't always the best ones, and we refuse to limit ourselves to the least common denominator in what we write and publish.

We're small and agile enough that we can exist in the spaces between the giants. In fact, we think that's where most of the exciting stuff is happening. We dig independent media. To the greatest extent possible, we work with people who share our values. If what we publish can make even the tiniest of difference, we've accomplished what we've set out to accomplish.

Starting in 2010, some of our titles will be published as an imprint of PM Press.

Tofu Hound Press was founded in 2005, and named for the two dogs who come running every time they hear us open a package of tofu. Of course we oblige, and think of it as an inexpensive royalty for using their story as our name.

Find out more at www.tofuhoundpress.com.

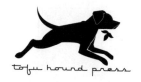

ABOUT PM PRESS

PM Press was founded at the end of 2007 by a small collection of folks with decades of publishing, media, and organizing experience. PM co-founder Ramsey Kanaan started AK Press as a young teenager in Scotland almost 30 years ago and, together with his fellow PM Press co-conspirators, has published and distributed hundreds of books, pamphlets, CDs, and DVDs. Members of PM have founded enduring book fairs, spearheaded victorious tenant organizing campaigns, and worked closely with bookstores, academic conferences, and even rock bands to deliver political and challenging ideas to all walks of life. We're old enough to know what we're doing and young enough to know what's at stake.

We seek to create radical and stimulating fiction and non-fiction books, pamphlets, t-shirts, visual and audio materials to entertain, educate and inspire you. We aim to distribute these through every available channel with every available technology — whether that means you are seeing anarchist classics at our bookfair stalls; reading our latest vegan cookbook at the café; downloading geeky fiction e-books; or digging new music and timely videos from our website.

PM Press is always on the lookout for talented and skilled volunteers, artists, activists and writers to work with. If you have a great idea for a project or can contribute in some way, please get in touch.

PM Press
PO Box 23912
Oakland, CA 94623
www.pmpress.org

FRIENDS OF PM PRESS

These are indisputably momentous times — the financial system is melting down globally and the Empire is stumbling. Now more than ever there is a vital need for radical ideas.

In the year since its founding — and on a mere shoestring — PM Press has risen to the formidable challenge of publishing and distributing knowledge and entertainment for the struggles ahead. With over 75 releases to date, we have published an impressive and stimulating array of literature, art, music, politics, and culture. Using every available medium, we've succeeded in connecting those hungry for ideas and information to those putting them into practice.

Friends of PM allows you to directly help impact, amplify, and revitalize the discourse and actions of radical writers, filmmakers, and artists. It provides us with a stable foundation from which we can build upon our early successes and provides a much-needed subsidy for the materials that can't necessarily pay their own way. You can help make that happen — and receive every new title automatically delivered to your door once a month — by joining as a Friend of PM Press. Here are your options:

> **$25 A MONTH:** Get all books and pamphlets plus 50% discount on all webstore purchases
> **$25 A MONTH:** Get all CDs and DVDs plus 50% discount on all webstore purchases
> **$40 A MONTH:** Get all PM Press releases plus 50% discount on all webstore purchases
> **$100 A MONTH:** Sustainer — Everything plus PM merchandise, free downloads, and 50% discount on all webstore purchases

More information at www.pmpress.org — click on the *Friends of PM* link.

Generation V

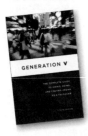

Going vegan is the single most important thing you can do if you want to get serious about animal rights. Yet, going vegan isn't always easy when you're young. You're living under your parents' roof, you probably don't buy your own groceries, and your friends, family, and teachers might look at you like you're nuts. So, how do you do it? In this essential guide for the curious, aspiring, and current teenage vegan, Claire Askew draws on her years of experience as a teenage vegan and provides the tools for going vegan and staying vegan as a teen. Full of advice, stories, tips, and resources, Claire covers topics like: how to go vegan and stay sane; how to tell your parents so they don't freak out; how to deal with friends who don't get it; how to eat and stay healthy as a vegan; how to get out of dissection assignments in school; and tons more. Whether you're a teenager who is thinking about going vegan or already vegan, this is the ultimate resource, written by someone like you, for you.

Alternative Vegan

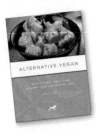

Taking a fresh, bold, and alternative approach to vegan cooking without the substitutes, this cookbook showcases more than 100 fully vegan recipes, many of which have South Asian influences. With a jazz-style approach to cooking, it also discusses how to improvise cooking with simple ingredients and how to stock a kitchen to prepare simple and delicious vegan meals quickly. The recipes for mouth-watering dishes include one-pot meals — such as South Indian Uppama and Chipotle Garlic Risotto — along with Pakoras, Flautas, Bajji, Kashmiri Biriyani, Hummus Canapés, and No-Cheese Pizza. With new, improved recipes this updated edition also shows how to cook simple to let the flavors of fresh ingredients shine through.

Lickin' the Beaters 2: Vegan Chocolate and Candy

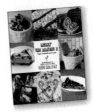

The beaters go on in *Lickin' the Beaters 2: Vegan Chocolate and Candy*, the second of Siue Moffat's fun vegan dessert cookbooks. Themed around the duality of dessert — an angel on one shoulder and a devil on the other — Siue takes chocolate candy and even ice creem (vegan alternative to ice cream) head-on with quirky illustrations, useful hints, and a handy "Quick Recipe" indicator to make using this book simple and amusing.

Recipes include old favorites such as Carmel Corn, Salt Water Taffy, Pralines, Cookies, Cakes, and Fudge, as well as some brave new gluten-free recipes like Fabulous Chocolate Torte and Toll-Free Chocolate Chip Cookies.

Cook, Eat, Thrive: Vegan Recipes from Everyday to Exotic

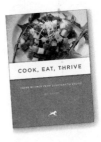

In *Cook, Eat, Thrive*, Joy Tienzo encourages you to savor the cooking process while crafting distinctive meals from fresh, flavorful ingredients. Enjoy comfortable favorites. Broaden you culinary horizons with internationally-inspired dishes. Share with friends and family, and create cuisine that allows people, animals, and the environment to fully thrive.

Drawing from a variety of influences, *Cook, Eat, Thrive* features a diversity of innovative vegan dishes, ranging from well-known favorites like Buttermilk Biscuits with Southern Style Gravy and Barbecue Ranch Salad to more exotic fare like Palm Heart Ceviche, and Italian Cornmeal Cake with Roasted Apricots and Coriander Crème Anglaise. With planned menus for all occasions, clear symbols for recipes that are raw, low-fat, soy-free, and wheat-free, and a section on making basics like seitan and non-dairy milks, *Cook, Eat, Thrive* is an essential book for anyone interested in cooking the very best vegan food. (Available winter 2010)

New American Vegan

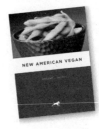

Across North America, people are looking to eat food that is not just more compassionate, but also healthier, more environmentally friendly and, most of all, tastes great. *New American Vegan* by Vincent J. Guihan breaks from a steady stream of vegan cookbooks inspired by fusion and California cuisines. Instead, the author goes back to his Midwestern roots to play a humble but important role in the reinvention of American cuisine while bringing the table back to the center of American life. Weaving together small town values, personal stories, 130 great recipes and hundreds of great ideas, *New American Vegan* delivers authentically American and authentically vegan cuisine that simply has to be tasted to be believed. Detailed, simple but elegant recipes also provide additional notes that explain how to take each recipe further, to increase flavor, to add drama to the presentation or just how to add a little extra flourish for new cooks and seasoned kitchen veterans. (Available spring 2010)

For more information visit www.tofuhoundpress.com and www.pmpress.org.